Menstrual & Pre-menstrual Tension

Well Woman series

jan de vries

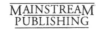
MAINSTREAM
PUBLISHING

EDINBURGH AND LONDON

First published in Great Britain in 1992 by
MAINSTREAM PUBLISHING COMPANY (EDINBURGH) LTD
7 Albany Street
Edinburgh EH1 3UG

Reprinted in 1998, 2001

A catalogue record for this book is available from the British Library

ISBN 1 84018 590 2

Typeset in 11/13 Palatino
Printed and bound in Great Britain by Cox and Wyman Ltd

Contents

Books available from the same author in the
By Appointment Only series:

Stress and Nervous Disorders (sixth edition)

Multiple Sclerosis (third edition)

Traditional Home and Herbal Remedies (fourth edition)

Arthritis, Rheumatism and Psoriasis (fifth edition)

Do Miracles Exist?

Neck and Back Problems (fifth edition)

Migraine and Epilepsy (fourth edition)

Cancer and Leukaemia (second edition)

Viruses, Allergies and the Immune System (fourth edition)

Realistic Weight Control

Who's Next?

Heart and Blood Circulatory Problems

Asthma and Bronchitis

Life Without Arthritis – The Maori Way

Books available from the same author in the
Nature's Gift series:

Body Energy

Water — Healer or Poison?

Foreword

by Gloria Hunniford

EVERY SO OFTEN along comes a natural communicator and broadcaster, who immediately builds up a worthwhile relationship with the listeners and viewers. Such a man is Jan de Vries. I have worked with him on various Radio 2 and television programmes since 1984, and the mailbag or phonelines have regularly been bursting with medical queries, which he has dealt with in excellent professional terms.

However, what has clearly emerged is the number of Well Woman medical problems. Therefore, as a result of the many questions on my programmes, Jan has embarked on the Well Woman series, starting with premenstrual and menopausal conditions, to be followed with books on the subjects of childbirth and pregnancy, mother and child, skin and hair conditions, and women's cancers. These books will answer in depth the many queries that we have had on the programmes and I do hope that this series of books will be of help with many of the presently common conditions.

A woman is the most reliable expert in her own health care.
—Dr Carolyn De Marco

1

Menstrual Tension

IN RECENT YEARS I seem to have been consulted more and more frequently by female patients seeking relief from physical and mental symptoms which are the direct result of menstrual or premenstrual tension. I wonder why so many women nowadays admit to suffering from these phenomena. Is it an urge to be in vogue by joining the ever-increasing number of sufferers or are these problems indeed more prevalent nowadays, or could it be that the taboo has finally been lifted and women, realising there is no longer any stigma attached to suffering menstrual and premenstrual tension, have become more inclined to discuss their symptoms openly? I have come to the conclusion that the answer is most likely a combination of the above assumptions. I am pleased that more women feel able to discuss these personal problems and no longer feel the need to repress them. I do not believe that menstrual or premenstrual tension can be regarded as a syndrome which has begun to occur only recently; it is far more likely that these symptoms are as old as humanity, but earlier generations would not discuss such problems, regarding them as essentially female and private.

The monthly cycle is dreaded by many women, and more than likely by equally as many husbands. There is little doubt that the family as a whole can suffer when the wife or mother is feeling out of sorts. Because she feels uptight, she is likely to be less tolerant towards the members of her immediate family and probably, as a direct result, her children will become more recalcitrant. Here we have all the makings of a confrontation, while the same circumstances at any other time of the month may not have caused any problems whatsoever.

From an article in a national newspaper I learned that menstrual tension supposedly affects 74 per cent of women of child-bearing age. Many women freely admit to a diminished sense of co-ordination and, to quote one example, volunteer that this is quite apparent in their driving ability at a certain time of the month.

It is acknowledged that marriages can come under stress because of tension at this time of the month, and unexpected aggression varying from a mild bad temper to violent outbursts are not unknown. Admittedly, these are some of the more extreme symptoms, which fortunately do not occur too frequently. On average, most women suffer a degree of irritability, depression, anxiety, inability to cope, bloatedness, and often a craving for sugar, even though these may be out of character at other times of the month. There are more symptoms that have been ascribed to this particular condition, symptoms that vary before, during and after menstruation. It is hardly surprising that such conditions account for an increasing number of psychiatric admissions and suicide attempts, many of which take place during the premenstrual phase.

However, let me be very clear. I do not want to create the impression that all extreme female emotions may be blamed regardlessly on a certain time of the month. Nor does it mean that women can claim indulgence for uncontrollable tempers on the ground of menstrual tension. Menstrual or premenstrual tension are phenomena that have been used by some as an excuse to include any kind of quarrelsome or obnoxious tendencies. Having said this, it may well be that such tendencies do only occur at certain times of the month, in which case some extra consideration will be required from the other members of the family. It is only too common for women to act uncharacteristically during periods of hormonal imbalance or change.

Let us take an overall look at the years of the average female fertility cycle. Menstruation usually starts during the early to mid teens and continues for approximately thirty to forty years. During this lengthy period the hormonal balance passes through various stages, according to age and circumstances. It is fairly common for periods to be irregular for teenagers during the early stages of menstruation. The cycle will regulate itself in the late teens or early twenties. A major hormonal change takes place during pregnancy, which is followed by a further change when the new mother is breastfeeding her baby. After such an experience the hormone level will eventually balance itself, naturally and in its own time. Towards the end of their fertile period many women experience a greater or lesser degree of irregularity in their menstrual cycle. This condition is called the menopause, and its onset indicates the end of the reproductive years.

Menstrual tension is often the result of undue pain experienced prior to or during menstruation and it is important to realise that much can be done to alleviate such side-effects. From the contents of this book you will learn that there is little or no need to suffer unduly during this time of the month.

Period pain — dysmenorrhoea — can be primary or secondary in nature. Primary dysmenorrhoea usually starts within a few months of a teenager's first menstruation and this condition is therefore most common among the under-25 age group. Abdominal cramps and pains can result in severe backache which can, however, be eased in a variety of ways. Please remember that there is no need to suffer such symptoms unnecessarily; so often women shrug their shoulders and say that it only lasts one or two days anyway, so why bother about it. Never forget that this condition can be avoided and effective relief can be obtained from some simple forms of alternative medicine.

Secondary dysmenorrhoea usually starts in later life, possibly caused by a dislocation of the vertebra, or a pelvic imbalance, or a narrowing between the discs. The result can be heavy menstrual bleeding — menorrhagia. It is estimated that an approximate blood loss of 80 ml is considered normal, but occasionally the bleeding can be excessive to the extent that the person concerned becomes anaemic. If such heavy blood loss occurs, every effort must be made to discover the cause, so that something can be done to remedy the situation.

Nothing is to be gained from overlooking the fact that although menstrual periods are a perfectly natural part of the female life, the female body is also designed for enjoyment and happiness. This may not be appreciated by the young teenager, who regards her first period as an awkward occurrence and a painful and bothersome curtailment of her physical freedom. This early stage can have a tremendous impact and sympathetic and sensible guidance is desirable, preferably given by the mother. She can try to approach this by pointing out the wondrous ways of nature, touching on fertility and pregnancy, and so explaining the essential and unavoidable monthly eruptions.

In this way the young girl will come to appreciate that the menstrual cycle and the changes that take place in a woman's body are perfectly normal and natural. They are a spontaneous and realistic biochemical and hormonal process which trigger physical and emotional responses. Because this topic was rarely discussed at home, and even less at school, it was shrouded in mystery by our parents' and grandparents' generations and it was often suggested that the side-effects were all in the mind. Nowadays, attitudes have changed and this taboo has been lifted, with the result that many aspects of menstrual tension have come to light.

In all fairness, therefore, it cannot be claimed that there has been a considerable increase in menstrual and related problems. At the same time, our increased knowledge on the subject enables us to alleviate and even eliminate many of the symptoms of these problems.

The myths surrounding menstruation are thankfully diminishing. During the Middle Ages it was believed that menstruation was a sign of sinfulness. It was inter-preted as a sign of female inferiority and in certain religious groups women were forbidden to take part in church services for the duration of their menstrual periods. In some civilisations this was an unwritten law, while the laws of other cultures were more specific as to the restrictions placed upon women during their period of "uncleanliness". Diverse rituals were adhered to throughout the world, stipulating how menstruating women should be isolated while they were "unclean" and subjected to all sorts of restrictions which affected their equality. Some of the effects were even attributed to witchcraft.

The medical profession has to take some of the blame because it previously refused to recognise these symptoms as the physiological effects of a natural occurrence. Fortunately, recent research has shown that it is quite possible for women to undergo a temporary but radical change in character as a result of hormonal changes. Within a short space of time some women can turn into aggressive, overpowering and bullying females, occasionally even with criminal tendencies. Some women will ashamedly admit in the privacy of my consulting rooms that they have beaten their husbands or that they have thrown crockery about, which under normal circumstances would be totally out of character. A chemical change in the hormones, prior to or during menstruation, is now recognised as being able to trigger a significant change in personality, causing a mercurial change in moods.

The effects are not only restricted to mental changes, since many more women report physical side-effects, such as asthma attacks, backache, tiredness, and even epileptic fits if there is already a tendency. When I try to explain such phenomena, women sometimes respond tritely: "Who are you to talk, because men get off scot-free!" I appreciate that it is sometimes difficult for a man to understand because the male sex hormones, which are also chemical messengers, remain on a much more even keel, whereas the levels of the female sex hormones, i.e. the luteinising hormone (LH) and the follicle-stimulating hormone (FSH), fluctuate greatly throughout the month. A slight imbalance of these hormones can cause problems. In Chapter 3, which looks at hormonal control, I will go into this in more detail, but at this point I can say that the pituitary gland — one of the smallest endocrine glands — is meant to stimulate the correct levels of oestrogen and progesterone production. These are two specific sex hormones, whose function is a strong contributory factor to menstrual problems.

It would be interesting to discover how nutrition affects the menstrual cycle and menstrual tension. In fact, we should look at the individual's whole lifestyle if we aim to improve control over the symptoms that can result from menstrual tension. We would do well to realise that although the effects of menstrual tension in the past were often considered as a curse, in reality they constitute a natural cyclic process that takes place in a woman's life. The average woman spends nearly half her lifetime in the menstrual cycle — anything between thirty and forty years between puberty and the menopause. This is the period that indicates fertility or the ability to conceive. In order to be able to produce children, a woman has to go through these phases and although fertility levels vary, according to statistics it has been calculated that approximately one pregnancy occurs per 900 cases of sexual intercourse.

The actual period of menstrual bleeding should never be too long. In fact, the average period should not exceed four or five days, and if it is longer medical help may need to be sought. Although there appears to be an increase in the incidence of menstrual problems, it has also become easier to curb or control excessive or critical effects, which was not possible for previous generations. The results of modern research and the removal of any stigma has given us the opportunity to counter any problems as and when they become apparent.

My primary reason for writing this book on the different kinds of menstrual stress is to explore some of the many methods that are now available to alleviate certain conditions. For instance, spasmodic dysmenorrhoea may be helped by specific exercises, as it is important to decrease the prostaglandin output and this can be achieved quite effectively with certain exercises. When a cell is damaged, chemical prostaglandin is released and in cases of spasmodic dysmenorrhoea it is important to prevent the excessive production of these chemical substances. Congestive dysmenorrhea usually occurs spontaneously and is characterised by severe abdominal pain which can persist for up to a week. At one time it was thought that water retention was an influential factor, but it is now thought that stress, worry and emotional upset are more likely to be the disturbing influences. It all comes down to hormonal imbalance.

Fybroids, abnormal tissue and possibly misplaced cells can all contribute towards menstrual tension. Such possibilities need to be checked and if there is any reason to suspect that such influences may exist you must seek the help of a qualified practitioner in order to obtain a correct diagnosis and treatment for any irregularities.

From experience, many of my female readers will agree that one of the major problems during the menstrual cycle is premenstrual tension and we will look more closely at this syndrome in the next chapter.

2

Premenstrual Tension

PREMENSTRUAL TENSION or premenstrual syndrome — PMT or PMS — is a hormonal imbalance which manifests itself through a variety of symptoms. Physical, mental and emotional problems can be experienced through symptoms such as fatigue, emotional instability, aggression, anxiety, depression, stress, tension, lack of concentration, confusion, fluid retention, headaches and asthmatic sinus problems.

Perhaps understandably, PMT is sometimes described as a "Jekyll and Hyde" condition and the only way to find out if PMT is at the root of the problem is to carefully record any symptoms together with the dates on which they occurred. If the symptoms recur in a cycle, it is fairly safe to conclude that the person concerned is subject to PMT.

Research suggests that 30–40 per cent of menstruating women suffer premenstrual tension and, indeed, some women experience very severe symptoms. Premenstrual tension may manifest itself at earlier or later stages in life, but for all who experience it, the diagnosis is the same — a hormonal upheaval. To learn more about the personal problems related to menstrual symptoms requires careful consideration. The timing of certain symptoms, and how this relates to ovulation and menstruation, should be monitored, if for no other reason than to understand what is happening in the body and mind. In this way at least the sufferer can be forewarned and will be better able to cope. It is no good losing confidence or shutting yourself away. Although premenstrual tension can be a very debilitating problem it can be overcome. Nothing is to be gained by denying its existence; it is much more sensible to recognise the problem and then look for help.

Some people still attach a stigma to premenstrual symptoms, yet they affect all women irrespective of class, age or colour. The media has helped to counter this by drawing greater attention to this previously almost unacknowledged syndrome. It is generally thought that nine out of ten women will at some time experience such symptoms; part of the problem is that the range and degree of patients' symptoms vary enormously.

I remember one patient who hesitantly informed me of tenderness and swelling of the breasts and then, gaining courage, she continued by listing weight gain, insomnia, abdominal bloating and greatly variable patterns in her sexual appetite. She desperately wanted me to agree that all these symptoms could not possibly be ascribed to PMT as her doctor had diagnosed. She was convinced that this was impossible and that there must be another cause. At the end of the consultation I had to tell her that I was in full agreement with the diagnosis her doctor had reached. I had no doubt that her problems were due to PMT. Together, we worked out a course of treatment which she followed carefully, and afterwards she admitted that both her doctor and I must have been right in our diagnosis, because the positive results of the treatment programme were clearly evident. Women should not worry that by acknowledging these problems they will be labelled a hypochondriac, because premenstrual syndrome has very real physical and psychological symptoms.

Many women would find it beneficial to spend a little more time and pay a little more attention to themselves during these times. Some positive consideration and understanding of how our bodies work will often reduce the symptoms almost immediately.

It should go without saying that health is and will always be a major issue and that without good health it is impossible to live and enjoy life to the full. I read some interesting facts and statistics in a report produced by the manufacturers of "Ladycare" products. From this report I learned that 48 per cent of the total British population and 42 per cent of the British workforce is female. The aim of this report was to demonstrate the living conditions for some women, how they conduct their lives, and the pressures to which they are subjected. I was rather surprised to learn that 92 per cent of the women surveyed believed that they should take responsibility for their own health, 33 per cent were worried about breast cancer and 30 per cent live in fear of cervical cancer. Medication alone was not considered an effective solution to health problems and 58 per cent actually agreed that too much medication was taken.

The largest ratio of women who complained of lack of energy, painful periods and premenstrual tension was found to be in the age group of 25–39 years. Also in this group, many admitted to suffering considerable stress. The 40–49 age group appeared to have more energy, but tended to worry about the menstrual cycle and how they would cope with the inevitable menopause.

Women over the age of fifty were slightly less worried about the menopause but tended to be more concerned about osteoporosis.

In this report it also became apparent that the type of problems experienced during the menstrual cycle seemed to change with age. The 25–39 age group suffered significantly more PMT (41 per cent of the total) than the 18–24 group (24 per cent). However, more younger women experienced painful periods (30 per cent against 21 per cent in the next age group), and stress and cystitis affected the younger age group more than any of the other groups.

Women who feel stressed complain more about PMT and lack of energy than women who are only slightly stressed or not at all. Those who feel dissatisfied with life also tend to complain of sleeplessness, severe lack of energy and an increase in the incidence of PMT, according to the report. It is felt that one third of all women smoke because of this stress problem. Unfortunately, more young women smoke than in any other age group, and surprisingly only 1 per cent of the smokers surveyed agreed that they were addicted. Similarly, more young women admitted to drinking alcohol on a regular basis than those in any other age group. In general, the answers in the survey pointed to the conclusion that the natural bodily functions seemed to cause little or no concern to the majority of women during their life cycle. They seemed to cope well with menstruation, pregnancy and childbirth. However, the experience or the expectation of premenstrual tension and the menopause seemed to cause considerable anxiety and discomfort.

The most frequently mentioned symptoms seemed to be emotional imbalance, i.e. inexplicable mood changes (83 per cent) and sudden onsets of depression and crying spells (57 per cent). Emotional instability is exacerbated by a bloated feeling, headaches and increased appetite, or a craving for chocolate or sugar. It was quite remarkable to see that according to this survey many problems were blamed on stress. It seemed that work was the main cause of stress and one third of the women with children claimed to worry more about them than about any other single factor. It was generally agreed that being able to talk about their feelings and problems appeared to be the most beneficial way of coping with stress. Financial problems were mentioned as the overriding stress factor by 16 per cent.

In summary, it was concluded that stress was caused by work, lack of money and day-to-day living, and many of the women felt that they would like the opportunity of sharing their problems with other women who would be able to recognise the symptoms. Surprisingly, though, few women rely on medication and only 3 per cent admitted to taking tranquillisers.

Diet, however, is of the greatest importance, as many women respond to a craving for chocolate, sugar and refined carbohydrates by indulging themselves. Unfortunately, eating vast amounts of refined carbohydrates and sugar is not the answer. During interviews with women in my own clinic I hear expressions of envy for those lucky patients that do not suffer from premenstrual tension. Many women compare premenstrual tension to living in a nightmare. I have also been told that I am to be envied, solely because I belong to the male of the species and I live in a male-dominated world, where premenstrual tension is often dismissed as hypochondria or neurosis. A lot of these women who come to me are sincerely worried about the possible effects of prescribed medication from their general practitioners, i.e. a hormone-based drug. Most would much rather help themselves with a natural remedy such as vitamin B_6. My reaction often disappoints them, because this is not really a satisfactory solution. Premenstrual syndrome, which is caused by a hormonal imbalance, deserves careful attention.

A well-known researcher in this field, Dr Guy A. Abrahams from California, has been investigating PMT for many years and has identified several types of premenstrual syndrome. He called these PMS-A, PMS-H, PMS-C and PMS-D, and has defined the symptoms of each as follows:

PMS-A: anxiety, nervous tension, mood swings and irritability;
PMS-H: hormonal weight-gain, bloating, swelling and breast tenderness;
PMS-C: craving for specific foods and sweets, headaches, heart-pounding, tiredness, dizziness and fainting;
PMS-D: depression, forgetfulness, crying spells, confusion and sleeplessness.

Dr Abrahams has reached some very interesting conclusions. The diet of women diagnosed as suffering from PMS-A symptoms appeared to be lacking in vitamin B_6 and magnesium. For women with the PMS-H diagnosis the case was more complicated; here he concluded that the problem was aggravated by a combination of stress, lack of magnesium and vitamin B_6, and a craving for sugar. The women in the PMS-C category exhibited deficiencies of specific nutrients such as essential fatty acids. The PMS-D symptoms were attributed largely to environmental factors, deficiencies of certain vitamins and minerals and a dietary imbalance.

In the light of his findings and as a means of self-help Dr Abrahams advised the following guidelines:

—healthy eating;
—careful examination of the vitamin, mineral and trace element intake;
—avoidance of stress;
—reduction of the intake of sweet foods;

—use of low-fat dairy produce;
—drastic reduction in the intake of coffee, alcohol and animal fats;
—discontinuation or severe reduction in nicotine consumption.

It is extremely important to understand that we are not dealing with a purely physical problem but that we are up against a combination of physical and mental symptoms which ought to be considered holistically. There is little to be gained by trying to control such symptoms with drugs alone, unless all aspects of the problems have been considered. The overriding stress factor which became apparent from the survey mentioned above has a direct effect on the hypothalamus and the pituitary gland, which in turn affect the ovaries and the sex hormones — the oestrogen and the progesterone production. All the endocrine glands are affected and involved in one way or another and in Chapter 3, which looks at hormone control, I will deal with this in more detail.

The premenstrual symptoms usually occur a few days or a week prior to menstruation. Yet they can also occur during the time of ovulation, that is, mid-cycle. The term premenstrual syndrome covers a very wide subject and treatment is always required when a woman becomes quite powerless to ignore the symptoms. Over the many years I have been in practice, I have often been asked whether I really understand this subject; more often than not I have been challenged, accusingly: "What do you really know about it — being a man." I can immediately respond by informing whoever has asked me that I have a wife and four daughters, and therefore PMT is a subject with which I have grown familiar, and about which I have learned plenty. I have lived closely with such problems and I have studied them in an attempt to learn how I can best help those women who suffer from PMT.

I am well aware that there can be many causes of premenstrual tension and over the years I have mediated between married partners, stressing the need for understanding and consideration. Marriages have been threatened because of difficulties in relationships, lack of understanding, problems at work, or problems with children, or perhaps because of general stress, lack of sleep, or even the use of the contraceptive pill, lack of exercise, resentment, unemployment, or poor dietary management. Any of these factors may influence the PMT condition.

"Am I suffering this alone or do other women have similar problems?" is another question I am often asked. The women who ask this question can easily be reassured because there are no boundaries to these problems. The consequences are suffered by women universally. It is more than likely that these problems have been present for centuries but they appear to have become more prevalent in recent decades, probably due to the more stressful conditions we live in and the greater attention paid to these problems by the media. The only way to try and overcome such problems lies in a holistic approach. The confusion must be cleared away and once a correct diagnosis has been reached and the correct category has been ascertained, a course of treatment can be decided upon.

The excellent book written by Dr Katherine Dalton, *Once a Month*, contains charts which enable the individual to determine which category of premenstrual symptoms she suffers from. I can earnestly recommend this book to the reader as it contains much useful advice on how to deal with PMT.

The severity of premenstrual tension may fluctuate, but the individual is not helped by being advised that she will have to learn to live with it. This attitude on the part of practitioners has caused untold harm and I have seen many severely depressed patients, among them a considerable number with suicidal tendencies. This is totally unnecessary because once the necessary action has been taken the emotional instability which can so easily get out of hand and lead to chronic depression and even to suicide can be avoided.

Lack of concentration or excessive tiredness is another problem which may strike a woman at particular times of the month. Premenstrual tiredness frequently leads to a decrease in ability and lack of concentration, and can have a devastating effect on examination results. It has often been claimed to be the cause for failing one's driving test.

Premenstrual irritability or aggression can present very difficult situations. For instance, with one of my daughters, who is normally the most placid, gentle and wonderful person, I would know immediately without her telling me when her period was due. The change in her attitude and character would be obvious and would express itself in an uncharacteristic irritability and impatience, and often an aggressive approach towards her schoolwork.

This trend is not only noticeable among younger women but among adult women too. They wonder why they feel so depressed and sometimes even spiteful. Uncharacteristically, they may shout at their families and, without knowing the cause for their unusual behaviour, they have taken to tranquillisers and anti-depressants. Little do they know that this course of action usually constitutes a case of jumping out of the frying-pan into the fire. I always feel sorry when it comes to this, because to me it is such a ruthless way of dealing with a problem that could be solved so much more efficiently by a more gentle method.

In my work with prisoners I have investigated how female prisoners with serious criminal records tend to behave during the build-up towards their menstrual periods. The results of these studies were remarkable and afforded me a better insight and greater understanding towards the individual. In many cases I found a relationship between the crime committed and their mental behaviour and outlook at a certain time of the month. My findings in this context lead me to stress the point that premenstrual syndrome should be treated holistically. By paying attention to the language of our bodies much can be learned and many problems may be solved before they get out of hand. Understanding this unspoken language will lead us towards an appreciation of the mental factors that are involved. By adopting a positive approach and conscious action one can deal effectively with such problems as and when they occur.

With this in mind, my advice must be to identify the problems experienced, make a chart and apply some of the advice given in the following chapters where it is applicable. Unfortunately, many PMT sufferers have this unbelievable problem of insecurity or lack of self-esteem. To outsiders it may not be so obvious, particularly when this only manifests itself at certain times of the month. It often demonstrates itself in insecurity, excessive sensitivity and emotional upset. These symptoms will transmit a body language which most probably will induce a negative feedback. Decide to tackle this problem with a positive approach: review your diet, follow a pattern of regular exercise and relaxation and attempt to reduce your workload. This is the time to join in social events. Women must realise that because they are affected by such exclusively female problems there is no need to feel less valuable than members of the opposite sex.

It saddens me that in certain parts of the world where I have worked the spirit of inequality among the sexes is still very apparent. Even though we live in a so-called "liberated" society, never forget that we should expect our doctor or practitioner, our husband or a friend to listen when we have a problem. It is your right to be able to choose what kind of treatment you would like to receive. As a female you have the right to choose whether to produce a baby, which is a treasure for many, and if the price for that ability is having to go through the menstrual cycle, so be it. If it wasn't for the menstrual periods, the chance of pregnancy would not exist. Not only do you have these rights, you also have the responsibility to learn to interpret the language of your body and to get to know and understand your body correctly, to reduce the amount of stress in your life and to look after your own health. You may be assured that there are ways to overcome the emotional conflicts which can drag you down on such a regular basis.

When we look at the other side of premenstrual symptoms we will find that some women, because of relatively minor changes, have gained an increased energy level, increased creativity or sexual drive because they have managed to exert control over all those typically female symptoms with the help of a well-balanced diet, the use of vitamins, minerals and trace elements, essential fatty acids, exercise and some positive thinking. The power of thought — especially positive thought — has an important bearing on a problem such as PMT.

Understanding our thought processes still tends to confuse us. Yet it really is simple. The conscious system covers every item of the body, from our brain to the soles of our feet. Yes, we even think with our liver, our ovaries or our stomach. If we are conscious, we think, but when unconscious, we are unable to think. Many of our teachings have been contrary to reason, such as the power of the mind, mind over matter, the power of the brain, which enables people to do such wonderful things. The brain is merely an organ, the same as our stomach, our endocrine system or our liver; it is controlled by a conscious system and especially the endocrine system, which is the subject of the next chapter. The brain is not the master, nor does it control the body. If even one endocrine gland is out of balance or order, then disharmony will result. The slow response of a torpid liver retards the action of the body, causing the emotions to become depressed. When your head is aching until you cannot see straight, then the question is: who is the master — the brain or another vital organ? The brain acts in accordance with the emotional transmissions from the conscious system, therefore when the conscious system becomes dull and lazy, the brain refuses to work, or becomes lethargic. There are brains within brains and cells within cells, but in truth there is but one mind in which all things exist.

Accurately speaking, man does not have three minds, nor does he even have one mind used solely for the purpose of storing knowledge, which can make life difficult. This is the reason why highly intelligent people are often impractical and lacking in common sense. Our thought processes are very complex. Because of the benefit of adopting a positive attitude towards problems such as menstrual or premenstrual tension, I would like to say a little more about the brain function, which will give the reader a better understanding of the function of the endocrine system, which controls the hormonal balance. Any disruption in that hormonal balance is likely to influence the PMT symptoms.

Just as there is a connection from the eyes, ears, nose and tongue to different parts of the brain, it is a fact that all other parts of the human anatomy have a connection with various cells of the brain. This may give us a slightly clearer idea of the many aspects to be considered in the actual functioning of our body.

Our thinking faculties may be divided into three different parts: objective, subjective and subconscious. Our thinking is transferred from a universal mind to any one of the three divisions of our brain. Our thoughts, actions and deeds depend greatly upon the action on our conscious system by the brain. If an organ or part of our body is not functioning properly it is likely to interfere with the communication from our conscious system to our brain causing heavy, lethargic thinking. Our blood, being the motor power of our body, is responsible for the action of our conscious system materially. We think according to the emotions of our body. If the circulation within the brain is interfered with because of a crooked neck or shoulder, or the atlas is out of place, or a bone in the skull is out of alignment, this will impose pressure upon the brain and will retard the action of even the heart of our conscious system, because the connection will have been disturbed. In many cases such a condition may lead to disorder, and often we do nothing, we merely wonder. The result could well be a failing memory, or mental lethargy, and the whole body will feel below par, creating a peculiar sensation throughout the whole system.

The fact is that undue interference has brought pressure to bear on the conscious system and has retarded the action of thought. I have enlarged on this phenomenon because in the next chapter we will see that with positive thought and action, and the use of colour, the symptoms of premenstrual syndrome can be controlled. We have to try to understand the action of the brain. It is very easy to sit in a quiet place and note the action of the mind as it passes from one portion of the brain to another.

It will help us if we can understand the functions of the three divisions: the objective thought occurs in the frontal part of the brain; the subconscious action occurs in the lower back part of the brain. These two parts are thought-conveyors and have a direct connection with the action of the subjective part of the brain. This last part seems to act in a similar way to the reverse gear of a car. When we think ahead and plan into the future, the thought transpires in the objective part of the brain. When we begin to think of the past, the subjective or central part of the brain then acts as the reverse gear of a car and relays the action of thought to the subconscious part of the brain. Thus, as our trend of thought changes from the future to the past, we feel a direct action in the subjective part of the brain.

A very good test of this action may be accomplished by sitting and looking into space without any object being visible to obstruct the view. We may look at a cloud or the moon and observe its shape and *colour*. This will cause the objective part of the brain to act. Then pay strict attention to the feeling and emotion of the brain as it changes from the objective to the subconscious. Slowly change the position of thought by thinking back to your childhood days. Think of some event that happened when you were seven or eight years old, or think of some of your playmates in your early days, and as the thought changes from the objective to the subconscious, you will feel the movement in the subjective part of the brain. After the playmates of your early life have entered into your train of thought, slowly move the action of your thought back to the objective part of the brain, looking again into space. As this takes place you will again notice the action in the subjective part of the brain. Brain, mind and thought will experience many different bodily influences that can and will interfere with our thinking. Various parts of our body have a direct connection with the brain. Pressure or disturbances are relayed to the brain from defects in the different parts of the body.

A small distance behind the subjective top of the brain there is even a section that connects with our toes. Let us take the big toe, for example. If it has an ingrown toenail, this pressure on the nerve will cause confusion in the brain. If we have aches and pains in the small of our back, then confusion arises in the subconscious part of the brain. Hence the reason that aromatherapy and reflexology are so important in the treatment of premenstrual problems.

Let us consider the sections that make up the brain: a fluid encased in small tissue sacs, which are surrounded by bones, i.e. the skull. The skull is divided into separate parts joined together with elastic fibre. If different sections of the skull move out of position, they will exert pressure upon the little sacs containing the fluid of the brain and this will affect many parts of the body. This explains why I have included a chapter on cranial osteopathy in this book, as this method of treatment will have a positive influence on PMT problems.

A disaligned skull may interfere with any natural talent that humanity is entitled to exercise. If the temporal position of the skull is out of alignment, it is very easily detected: move your hands slowly over the skull and you will discover a groove or uneven surface of the skull. If this is the case with the parietal bones, pressure on the nervous system of the entire body will result, causing a person to worry. If the frontal bones have moved far enough out of position to bring pressure on the frontal part of the brain, it interferes with intelligence. If the lower division of the skull in the back of the head — the occiput — moves down, even the slightest bit, it will cause pressure on the mastoid gland and this will interfere with the hearing. The same condition may cause serious eye strain.

Thus, if pressures are brought to bear on different parts of our brain, they cause interference with our thinking. If we have a correct understanding of our thinking and hearing we can use the mind to a great extent. There is but one mind that is universal and it passes through the three divisions of our brain. If the brain is clear of bodily pressures and any interference within the nervous system, we can translate the universal mind into valuable thinking as the mind passes through the translator which is located in the frontal part of our head. We may translate from this mind some very valuable thoughts which bring us the information that we have been seeking for years. Many things that seemed to be confusing and hard to understand will be made plain to us by clear thinking. But this demands clear action of the brain. In order to have this clear action, we must have a clear brain. In order to have a clear brain, we must have a body that is functioning properly, free from aches and pains. Our conscious system must be free from depression, free of all the problems which are recognised as part of the PMT syndrome. Therefore if we have a real reconnection with mind, body and soul, we can think correctly, both physically and mentally, and we have to be careful when we translate the mind into thought. For example, if the imagination builds up in the subconscious part of the brain, a picture of jealousy, there will develop a yellowish-brown spot on different parts of the body. When a view is visualised in goodness and projected to all parts of the body, you will achieve perfect harmony. This is really the first step to end the monthly misery of PMT.

It is known that 40 per cent of women seek medical help to find relief from these symptoms, and because there are approximately 150 different symptoms relating to PMT, it is very difficult to pinpoint exactly what is going on. Therefore, in order to explore the causes of menstrual and premenstrual tension, the multitude of symptoms needs to be categorised and therefore further research and investigation must take place in order to find out the exact problem. It is known that many women still treat themselves and probably suffer unnecessarily some of the symptoms if this is not dealt with properly.

There are many ways to ease or overcome PMT and I intend to deal with many of them in this book. Even the smallest gland in the body may cause problems or perhaps could influence the hormonal balance negatively. Take, for example, that small gland called the pineal gland. It is the light receptor, or perhaps the aerial to the cosmic energy, and if disturbed it can affect the entire body. If our bodies were computers the pineal gland would control much of the software that triggers and programmes many brain functions. For more than twenty years scientists and researchers have been trying to work out how the pineal gland manages, for instance, to turn darkness into a chemical form. In frogs, for example, the gland itself is a light sensor, but in man the process is much more sophisticated and intricate. Light and darkness are detected by the eyes. Information travels to the spinal cord, from the optic nerve to the sympathetic nerve and the signal is carried back to the pineal gland, which is working twenty-four hours a day. A whole unexplored world has been opened up with questions relating directly and indirectly to the pineal gland. In the next chapter we will look for some further explanations.

3

Hormonal Control

"HOW CAN YOU expect me to believe that by wearing a different coloured skirt or dress I could end my premenstrual tension? I have suffered from it for years and now you are trying to tell me that by changing the colour of my clothes I could put a stop to it."

It wouldn't be the first time I have heard female patients utter such reactions with clear disbelief. Can colours really have any relevant impact on whether or not menstrual symptoms are experienced? I can assure you that with some simple adjustments the conditions can be reversed. Later in this chapter I will explain how colours can be used to influence favourably certain health conditions, including menstrual or premenstrual tension, but before I do, let us have a look at the endocrine system.

The pertinent question is how much do we know about the endocrine system? Even endocrinologists admit that there are still many questions to which, as yet, we

36

have not found a satisfactory answer. I believe that a holistic approach to the endocrine problem, or to what is often referred to as hormonal control, would give us a much clearer insight, and so a better chance to get to the root of the problem. Such an approach is applicable to physical and mental issues. The founder of homoeopathy, Dr Samuel Hahnemann, would always consider three factors: the mind, body and soul. One of the reasons that menstrual symptoms along with many other female complaints appear to be more prevalent today is because the endocrine system is put under such severe pressure by a wide range of environmental and stress-related factors. In this context we must take into account poor dietary habits, atmospheric influences and some of the tools and machines we use in order to make life easier. These are not always beneficial to the endocrine system, which is extremely delicate and sensitive and responds to very minor vibrations, which are capable of effecting a change in the harmony of this intricate and diverse system.

There are seven endocrine glands and there are also seven layers of light receptors in the retina of the eye. Moreover, there are seven colours in the solar spectrum as well as seven scale steps in a musical octave. All these groups require harmony for the maintenance of a healthy and happy lifestyle. If only one of the endocrine glands is out of balance, they all will suffer to a certain extent; if only one is out of tune, none of the others will function to optimum ability. In our attempt to find perfect harmony I often explain that, although they may be small, these seven glands require great respect. Compare the endocrine glands to an orchestra which is expected to play in harmony, and you will understand that these glands should exist and function in harmony if we are to obtain the best from life.

Some of these glands are no bigger than a pinhead or a small vitamin tablet and yet they exert a powerful influence over the entire body. By looking at each one in turn, we can begin to appreciate how and why it is so important to consider the endocrine glands when looking for a means to overcome menstrual or premenstrual tension. Some simple advice may enable the reader to make a change and tune back into harmony.

Although reflexology is occasionally ridiculed, the more we learn about the endocrine system, the more we will realise that reflexology can be of benefit. It has been determined that by exerting pressure on certain parts of the big toe the whole endocrine system can be positively influenced through the pineal gland and the pituitary gland. By exerting pressure to areas on the heel we can affect the genitals. An osteopath, by working on the cranium, may influence the pituitary, the hypothalamus, the thyroid or even the pineal gland. It is also true that we can positively or negatively influence the endocrine system with our diets management. A simple herbal remedy can also bring about a considerable change. It is amazing to hear women who have suffered for years from menstrual symptoms extolling the virtues of what, to all intents and purposes, was only a minor adjustment but has brought about a dramatic change in their life.

In this book it is not my intention to explain in detail all the complexities of the hormonal secretions that take place in our bodies, or to overload you with details of the relationship between the endocrine glands. The endocrine system is widely acknowledged as being very complex and yet our actions and lifestyle can be decisive in the fine tuning of these glands, particularly at certain times of the monthly cycle. The two endocrine glands which are of major importance in the menstrual cycle are the pituitary and the pineal glands. In her excellent book, *What's Wrong With You?*, my good friend Dorothy Hall refers to the pineal gland as "the composer" and equates the pituitary gland to "the conductor". I like these expressions because they convey to us the importance of the role that these glands perform in our body.

Let us take first the pituitary gland — the conductor. It is the function of this gland to control hormonal release and distribution and to maintain the balance in the hormonal household. A further important factor is that the "conductor" exerts control and influence over all the other glands, and for this reason must be regarded with respect. Some of the endocrine glands are so sensitive that conditions can change relatively quickly. Such changes can be brought about or influenced by certain foods we eat or even by negative thoughts. In early medical books the pituitary gland was often referred to as the "gland of wisdom". It is widely considered as an extremely responsive gland and even minor attention or consideration given to the pituitary gland will produce a positive result. Glandular hormones pass directly into our bloodstream and in combination they are likely to renew the life and vigour of the body. In the absence of any one of these hormones, the blood immediately becomes unbalanced.

In the case of the pituitary gland we know that more than one hormone is produced. Rather than dazzle you with complicated names, I will just skip through them. As long as we understand their function, we will appreciate their importance. There is the hormone that influences the regulation of the blood pressure, helps to rebuild blood vessels and renews any veins that have been destroyed by tubercular conditions. Another hormone controls the cerebrospinal fluid of the spinal column. The same hormonal secretion maintains the secretion of urine and stimulates lactation in the mammary glands, when they are active. A further hormone exerts a stimulating effect on the tissues of the smooth muscles of the body, causing contraction of the uterine muscles for example, and is essential for the bladder and reproductive organs. The pituitary gland also secretes a substance which plays a part in the release of steroids from the adrenal glands, and so regulates the growth of the skeleton. When the pituitary gland is inactive, the face, hands and feet often swell as a result of fluid retention. During a period of inactivity the gland may also increase in size, exerting pressure on the optic nerve and causing a certain type of blindness. Bloating of the face may be the cause of yet further disturbances in the head, which may result in headaches. The temporary increase in size of the pituitary may hinder the circulation, causing lightheadedness or dizzy spells, which in turn can cause a person to stagger or lose their sight temporarily. In summing up some of the functions and responsibilities of the pituitary gland, I have tried to give you an indication of the tremendous role this "conductor" plays in the glandular orchestra.

Now we move on to the work of the "composer", i.e. the pineal gland. Although this gland is undoubtedly of tremendous importance, unfortunately relatively little is known about it and therefore it receives very little recognition in the medical world. The role of the pineal gland is underestimated, as is that of the thymus gland. The pineal gland is also known as the "aerial of the body". This "third eye" is open to influences of any kind. It is fascinating, yet also disturbing, to see the effects on the pineal gland of watching television. Kirlian photography enables us to see how the energy aura of the pineal gland is reduced by the influence of a television screen. The same applies to the visual display unit of a computer or word processor. Atmospheric influences also have a bearing on the well-being of the pineal gland.

Animals live much closer to nature and instinctively acknowledge the important functions of the pineal gland. Accordingly, animals have a larger, better developed and more active pineal gland than humans. Even in humans the size of the pineal gland varies according to lifestyle and responds to advantageous circumstances and influences, for example relaxing in the open air, quietly learning to understand oneself, or spending some time in meditation. I have seen among my immediate family how easily menstrually influenced depression can be lifted by listening to or playing a piece of music, quietly withdrawing to meditate upon something positive, singing a song, or going for a walk in the fresh air. These are all positive responses which allow the pineal gland to prosper, thus allowing the "composer" to direct all the other endocrine glands towards harmony.

This small gland is treated with more respect in the Far East than it is in our Western world, and we would benefit greatly from following their example. It can never be replaced by material substances and can only be restored by the cosmic chemistry — as it is the aerial for atmospheric influences. It is even capable of producing mineral substances of various kinds. Scientific tests have been conducted on the pineal gland with respect to its production of calcium phosphate and carbonate and magnesium phosphate.

In *Gray's Anatomy* we read that the pineal gland produces and stimulates seven different minerals in the human body and that its action is carried by the spinal column. The importance of magnesium and calcium is widely recognised in relation to menstrual symptoms. If the circulation in the spinal cord is obstructed, the pineal gland will become swollen or enlarged. This, in turn, will interfere with the function of the four main ventricles of the brain, which regulate the medulla in the brain and other bodily functions. Such an obstruction will also cause unnatural pressure on the optic nerves of the eyes and the auricular nerves of the ears, retarding their function. So, we see that the "composer", i.e.

the pineal gland, needs time for objective thinking and meditation before being able to compose a suitable piece of music for the endocrine orchestra to play!

The thyroid is yet another endocrine gland affected by today's stressful lifestyle. The two lobes of the thyroid are finely balanced and work together as well as individually. The Chinese teach their medical students to observe the condition of the hair, skin and nails, which provide a visible indication of thyroid efficiency. Similarly, arthritic conditions, especially hormonal arthritis which is more often found in younger women, are related to an inefficient thyroid function. In the course of my work I see many goitres and much instability of the thyroid, mostly caused by poor dietary management, or by drinking or smoking.

The thyroid hormones are very sensitive, which is why distressing emotional experiences such as a divorce, an unhappy relationship, jealousy or resentment, or unemployment can trigger a drastic negative influence.

I remember the dietician who came over from the Netherlands to work in our residential clinic in Scotland. She was a very sensible person and refused to take any drugs to treat her under-active thyroid; instead, she particularly chose to work in our clinic because it was situated on the coast. The sea air and good dietary management helped her to overcome her problem completely. She told me that at the time of her periods she used to experience severe menstrual problems and how these problems had been greatly reduced since she had settled in Scotland. We met again several years after she had left us and she was a much happier person and had not suffered any further thyroid problems.

More evidence of thyroid problems can be seen in the enormous number of people who struggle to keep their weight under control. Certainly the thyroid is an influential factor in cases of obesity, but there are also a number of herbal remedies that can assist us to regulate our weight.

A bloated feeling caused by fluid retention is one of the problems that can occur because of a thyroid condition. Therefore the advice in this book is directed towards improving the function of the thyroid. Specific measures for thyroid hormone adjustment are best talked through on an individual basis with a homoeopathic practitioner, a herbalist or a naturopath, who will advise on careful changes that are suitable for long-term treatment.

Goitre problems or a swollen neck sometimes result from conditions in the cervical region and in such cases cranial osteopathy will often help. Enlargement of the neck can also be caused by an over-active thyroid or possibly by a hormone imbalance relating to the pituitary gland which then interferes with the voice and throat. Dislocation of the bones situated between the shoulder blades may also be responsible for this condition and often the problems, which originated in the thyroid gland, can be relieved by some minor osteopathic manipulative treatment.

The thyroid gland produces different hormones which enter the bloodstream. If there is an enlargement of the neck caused by a thyroid condition, serious problems could result. If these hormones in the thyroid are prevented from leaving it, they could lead to an abnormal heart function which in turn could cause a rapid pulse. As the thyroid gland increases in size, it causes the eyeballs to protrude. The stress of the protrusion acts on the tear ducts so that tears appear with the slightest strain or aggravation. The thyroid gland is of greater importance than is realised by many who are supposed to be authorities in the field of physiology. In the medical world there are a great number of different and opposing views on this subject.

Each lobe of the thyroid gland has a connection with the veins in our neck. The blood passes back and forth through the thyroid gland, which acts as a filter, eliminating the detrimental hormones from the blood. When the hormones have been separated, they pass from the two large lobes, one on each side of our throat, into the heart. It appears that in these lobes a number of different hormones are produced. The main hormone resembles iodine and the other hormones contain a small percentage of sulphuric acid. But nature has equipped the thyroid with a hormone that is necessary for purifying the blood before it enters the heart. Sometimes this hormone will be brownish-red or grey-blue in colour, resembling the main substance of our lymphatic system. Connections from these glands extend down into the stomach or to the walls of the stomach. On the inside of the stomach are little assimilators resembling warts, whose task is to extract the nutrients that are essential for manufacturing our blood from the food in our stomach. When the action and duty of our body's glands are clearly understood they can be maintained in perfect functioning order and, when all carry out their ascribed tasks, they will provide every substance that is required to rebuild our body.

Many a brilliant career has been spoilt by the appearance of a goitre. Many individuals have lost much of their confidence and many of their friends, all because of this defect. Happy homes have been broken up by the upset a goitre has caused in the blood of an individual. It tends to make the individual irritable, dissatisfied and inclined to find fault. Other people are always thought to be doing the wrong thing. It destroys peace and rest at night. Over-stimulation by such a person causes excessive activity at times. A person is then easily influenced to do things that his better judgement may warn him not to do.

This toxic poison has a tremendous influence over the subconscious part of the brain, causing us to ignore and doubt other people and things, and establishes in us a great fear. It affects our kidneys and urinary organs and the impaired condition of the subconscious part of the brain creates many false desires and passions, often leading to the development of bad habits. The effect of this toxic poisoning on the calcium level in our body is such that it diminishes the vibrations that determine willpower, thus making it impossible for us to abstain from the things that we most detest. Again, the endocrine system cannot be viewed only from a physical point of view, and a positive mental outlook will help the thyroid gland in many ways.

Just below the thyroid, situated centrally behind the sternum in the upper chest, the thymus gland can be found. Unfortunately, this gland has been largely ignored because the medical profession believes it to have little or no value after the age of forty. It seems that by that age it has dwindled away to the size of a pinhead. Yet I believe that the thymus gland is one of the most important glands in the human body. We must not forget that it forms part of the total endocrine system and that interference with it may well lead to problems elsewhere.

I remember the case of one lady who had a myasthenia gravis. After lengthy deliberation she gave permission for an operation and her thymus gland was duly removed. As she lived nearby I had a good opportunity to study her behaviour and I was surprised how strangely this developed. She became almost a different person, which of course confirmed my conviction that the thymus cannot be regarded from only a physical point of view, but the mental aspect must also be considered. The immunity of this lady was also drastically affected. Recent scientific investigations by immunologists have shown that the occurrence of auto-immune diseases is linked to the condition of the thymus gland. Especially in the early stages of life, the condition of the thymus gland is often a decisive factor.

Latterly I have been involved in some scientific work with a cancer group and we have noticed the importance of the thymus gland when cancer and leukaemia have been diagnosed. A poorly functioning thymus gland will be influential in the functioning of the immune system and I firmly believe that much more investigation should be carried out into the efficient working of the thymus gland, which plays a part in maintaining the harmony of all seven endocrine glands.

At a conference I once heard the remark that the thymus gland is the seat of our life energy. Probably the best way to illustrate the truth of this is by giving the thymus gland a little nudge, when we will see how this revitalises our energy. There is also a very close relationship between the thymus gland and the reproductive organs throughout our life. In the Far East I was taught that the thymus gland not only acts as a filter, but that the gland can be influenced by love and understanding.

A throat congestion or a goitre may cause swelling in the thymus gland. Some famous singers have experienced serious problems with their throat, resulting in the loss of control of their voice, and often it appeared that this distress was caused by the impaired action of the thymus gland. This gland, which has a direct link with the blood, heart and spleen, is inhibited by the red corpuscles, proving its distinct connection with the veins and arteries of the body. Congestion of the thymus gland will influence the circulation and its various interactions, especially in the case of menstrual or premenstrual tension, and this possiblity ought, therefore, to be considered. Adjustment of the tissues of the gland will often result in improvement. In most of these cases we will find that the sixth and seventh cervical vertebrae are out of position, thus impinging on the action of the nerves and inhibiting the circulation to the thymus gland. When we acquire more knowledge of the thymus gland I am sure that we will be able to improve the general health of mankind. This minute gland that plays such a great part in the harmony of life deserves much more attention than it currently receives.

When we turn to the pancreas, we again find a very complex area where the metabolic system depends upon the thyroid and the adrenals. I often wonder why the incidence of diabetes has increased so dramatically in recent years and I am quite sure that it is because the pancreas suffers so badly as a consequence of today's lifestyle. Pancreatic enzymes and secretions are extremely important for the correct functioning of the body, hence the reason that I have chosen dietary management as the subject of the next chapter. After the liver, the pancreas is one of the most important organs in the metabolic system and although the pancreas is about twenty times lighter than the liver, this little gland situated above the navel and between the vertebrae has a very important function to perform. It actually has a dual purpose and by overloading it with the wrong kinds of food we can induce problems such as diabetes. When considering the pancreas we also come to understand why diet is so important during the menstrual and premenstrual periods, as the production of the correct enzymes and amino acids is essential in this monthly cycle. Small clusters found in the pancreas, reminiscent of berries, are little gland cells and it is vitally important that these cells function correctly. If not, diabetes may well occur. A little dietary adjustment is often sufficient to stimulate these cells into functioning properly.

This brings us to the adrenals and the reason why we often hear complaints of a bloated feeling occurring around the time of menstruation. The urinary system is linked to different functions: it not only eliminates the waste water from the system, but eliminates many of the broken down minerals and tissues from the body. When we speak of urinary organs, we are referring to the kidneys, ureter and bladder. This system constitutes a complicated network and draws the decomposed minerals from every part of our body, with the exception of the water that is eliminated through the sweat glands or pores of the skin. Of course, the bladder is the main reservoir for the water that remains after the body has taken what it needs. Waste material, which is nothing more than decomposed solids which have become liquified, is eliminated through the kidneys and other channels.

The inside of our kidneys is divided into several cavities and it is here that the waste material is filtered from the blood. Cell tissue in the kidneys also has an important task. A gland, called the adrenal or the suprarenal gland, is attached to each kidney, located immediately above and in front of the upper end of the kidney. These adrenal glands produce two or three kinds of hormones, some of which help to neutralise the substances as they enter the kidney and help to separate the broken down minerals from the blood. Then the kidneys filter out this refuse into two large tubes — the ureters — which extend down to the bladder at the lower extremity of the body. The hormones secreted by the adrenal glands stimulate the tissue and the action of our kidneys, if the glands are in perfect working order. They also stimulate the action of the blood as it leaves the kidneys and the blood conveys this stimulation to the heart.

The location for treatment of the adrenal glands is at about the seventh rib or just above the extreme lower end of the sternum. It may be helpful to remember that in our skin we have two million or more glands and the skin eliminates a certain percentage of the poison, or dead tissue, from our body. It is therefore necessary for us to keep our skin soft and pliable so that perspiration can leave the body freely, carrying with it the debris that has settled in the pores and this will relieve the kidneys of the overload frequently forced upon them.

The organism which is our body is mechanically woven together. For instance, there is a link between certain little cells in the kidneys and the duodenum and there are certain areas in the kidneys that relate to or are connected with different organs in the colonic areas, the suprarenal gastric and the pancreatic areas. Many organs in the body have a drainage canal leading to the kidneys. The various tissues are so interwoven that it is almost impossible to describe them.

The energy in the kidneys is provided from the spinal column, at the twelfth dorsal of the twelfth rib. The short rib is always considered the kidney area and if this bone happens to be out of position, it will affect the action of the kidneys and retard the action of the adrenal glands, thus depriving the kidneys of the valuable hormone produced by these glands. In many cases adrenaline is given under these conditions, as this medicine is supposed to replace the hormone that is produced by these glands. But again there are other, gentler ways to deal with it. It is very important that harmony reigns in this area because any emotional trauma, upset, stress or anxiety will immediately affect the kidneys and the adrenal glands.

We must consider carefully how best to help the kidneys and the adrenals by means of exercise and other methods in order to stimulate the production of adrenaline. I am often asked how I manage to work such long hours, and I am quite sure that my adrenaline operates in such a way that it keeps me going. The enthusiasm I have for my work is also a contributory factor, and is bound to influence the life force. Whenever someone experiences tiredness or lethargy, the adrenaline level is low. Serious problems may occur in cases of trauma, when the use of cortisone will be a last resort, as it only gives a temporary respite, and increases the chance of further and more serious problems.

Prevention is always better than cure. It is not always necessary to take extra progesterone in order to control a hormonal imbalance. Such a condition can sometimes be overcome with a simple vitamin preparation or a herbal remedy and in Chapter 5 we will read more about this.

Over-active adrenals are usually the result of poor dietary management. Frequently, especially among younger women, we can identify a hormonal arthritic condition, which has been allowed - to develop from an initial disharmony. The pituitary gland releases a hormone which sounds the alarm. This hormone travels in the blood until it reaches the two small glands that sit on our kidneys in the middle of the back — the adrenals. When the adrenals absorb this hormone, they too release different hormones, the chief of which is called cortisol, also known as cortisone. Messages are also transmitted from the nervous system and the hormone adrenaline is released. The presence of these adrenal hormones in the blood indicates that the whole body is under threat. The adrenals produce cortisol from the hormone deoxycortisol — DOC for short — which helps the body fight infection and damage by setting up an inflammation around bacteria or toxins and sealing them off, as in boils for example. So once again, we can see how correct dietary management is important, especially during the menstrual cycle and where menstrual problems are experienced. It is foolish to ignore the alarm signals: action should always be taken to prevent the situation recurring.

We now come to the last of the endocrine glands, the ovaries or the gonads, which are obviously of vital importance. The adrenals and the ovaries interrelate and are subjective to each other. The ovaries play an important role during the menstrual cycle. They are almost almond shaped and are positioned on either side of the uterus. The cervix, or neck of the womb, is like a little ball and is situated towards the back of the vagina. When the cervix begins to open a few days before ovulation, i.e. when the egg is released by the ovary, special cells in the cervix produce verticervical mucus, which allow the sperm to live during the journey to the uterus. When the menstrual blood passes through the cervix and flows into the vaginal canal, the muscular tube widens. The ovaries are the most important endocrine glands in the female. The hormones they produce include oestrogen and a group of related substances which make up the folicular hormone. The ovaries also produce progesterone, which is the corpus luteal hormone involved in menstruation. Any disturbance of the oestrogen and progesterone production will always cause irregularities in the menstrual cycle and other disturbances involving the female reproductive organs.

Hormones in general regulate and integrate the important activities of the body and they usually act directly on the tissues or organs controlling the activity of substances produced. They control the metabolism, the level of energy, the utilisation of sugar and the water balance; they regulate the alkaline/acid system and curb disturbances stemming from deficiencies. An excess production of even one hormone could lead to a total hormone imbalance. Each endocrine gland has a very delicate balance and disease or malfunction of any one can create a complete disarray of body functions.

If we now reconsider the seven basic scale steps of the musical octave, the seven layers of light receptors in the retina of the eye, or the seven colours in the solar spectrum, we are more likely to reach a better understanding of the endocrine system.

Firstly, we must consider the eyes and the sense of sight. The optic nerve, when it leaves the eyeball, travels to the centre of visualisation and imagination and to the cross-section of the medulla. The nerves branch out from this point, making their way to the spinal column. You will find that one pair connects to the third cervical, or between the third and fourth cervical vertebrae, which are situated in the middle part of the neck. From the third cervical the current will continue, down to the heart and stomach. We have three things to consider in relation to our sight: first there is the condition of our soul, next the condition of our stomach, and finally that of our circulation.

We will now return to the forehead or to the bridge of the nose for just a minute. When we place our thumb and forefinger on the bridge of the nose and the forehead we will see that the tension is leaving the eyes. The reason for the removal of this eye strain is the mineral passing from the hand to the centre of visualisation. Then the mineral travels down the nerves to the top bone of the spine — the atlas — because the mineral will automatically move the atlas back into its proper position, releasing the nerves, thus causing the strain and tension of the eyes to disappear.

Next, if you place the fingers on the back of the neck, on the middle bone between the shoulders and the skull, it is possible that you will find a sore point. Usually this is caused by a disc being slightly out of position. If the disc is completely misaligned, this may well have caused diminishing sight, or some other eye problem. With continuous treatment it is possible that the cervical disc will move back into place by itself, sometimes with the help of deep breathing. Many people have managed to regain their sight in this way. It is not unknown for people to be able to put aside their spectacles after manipulative treatment. It is therefore very helpful to practise some visualisation techniques, because when experiencing menstrual or premenstrual tension, positively visualising that it will soon pass may well help you along the road to recovery.

The seven layers of light receptors in the retina of the eye are important to the iridologist because so many functions of the body can be observed in the eyes. By using the eyes in a similar way to our other sense organs such as the ears, nose, mouth and tongue, they can serve as a useful diagnostic tool. Iris diagnosis is expedient because the iris reflects the condition of all the other systems in the body, and the eyes possess this built-in mechanism which indicates incoming light, frequency and colour. Any hereditary problems, for instance, can be identified through an abnormal discoloration in the eyes, and any changes connected to the monthly cycle will also be obvious in this way.

We are so colourfully made that each organ and each gland gives off its own unique translation of its function and chemistry in the brilliance of colour. Just reflect on how wonderfully man is composed! There are some 120 million rods — tiny receptors — in the eyes for perceiving light and translating it into electrical impulses. These impulses stimulate the pituitary gland, which in turn stimulates all the other glands. It is also fascinating to learn that the seven light waves correlate to the seven glands and their frequencies. Each gland generates an energy which is transmitted by powerful hormones to the tissues and nerves stimulating its specific action. Throughout the whole body colour variations reveal the characteristics of each tissue cell and a single vibration or change of tune can cause a deviation in colour.

In an interesting book called *Health and Light* I read that Africans did not know what arthritis was until the Americans introduced sunglasses. The green-tinted glasses filtered out the longer light waves resulting in an adrenal malfunction and consequently reducing their production of cortisone and other hormones. This explanation may seem odd, but it is impossible for us to divorce ourselves from the complete solar entity, simply because, by doing so, we could be inviting complications that are detrimental to our health. We can help our bodies best by appreciating the intricate design and the beauty of how we are made and then finally tuning in to this colourful solaria, which is as freely available to us as it was to the ancient civilisations who practised colour therapy in their own ways. Our forefathers learned to master the skills required to manufacture coloured glass. We have learned about cosmic light and radiation, and so the foundations of colour therapy were proven. This knowledge was acquired so that mankind could manipulate this cosmic energy with its vibrations and frequencies to suit its own individual needs.

I have spoken to many female patients who confided in me about their menstrual problems about a simple but marvellous therapy which has proved to be of great benefit, especially to those who have a regular monthly cycle. If, however, the periods are irregular, try to work out with the help of a chart if any pattern can be detected. About a week before the period is due, start wearing the colour of the pituitary gland — cyanogen blue. On the second day wear something violet; on the third day — green; on the fourth day — yellow; on the fifth day — orange; on the sixth day — orange-red and on the day before the period — red. The day after the period wear something greeny-blue, and you will feel great. The pituitary gland is well served by the cyanogen blue, the pineal gland by violet, the thyroid by green, the thymus by yellow, the pancreas by orange, the adrenals by orange-red, and the ovaries by red.

Because the above is a very unassuming piece of advice, I fear that to some people it may appear too simple to be effective or even contemplate, but even if you are sceptical, there can surely be no harm in trying. I can assure you that you will experience an astonishing improvement in harmony between yourself and nature and, as a bonus, you will gain in vital energy.

4

Dietary Management

I HAVE OFTEN been asked if it is true that certain foods can aggravate menstrual and premenstrual tension and if it is possible to be especially sensitive or allergic to certain foods during either the actual period of menstruation or the days immediately prior to it. There are several reasons for such questions because if the symptoms that are experienced are forgetfulness, emotional fragility, unusual weight gain or a distended stomach, there is the possibility of an allergic reaction to wheat, grains or yeast. Moreover, if the individual has a tendency towards *Candida albicans*, or thrush, the symptoms are likely to be ten times worse. Therefore, in a nutshell, the answer must be yes; dietary management *is* important in such conditions, as it is not unknown for wheat or wheat products to aggravate symptoms at this time of the month. In order to find out if an allergy is at the root of the problems, certain foods could be eliminated from the diet, one at a time.

Women who suffer from menstrual or premenstrual symptoms frequently complain of a bloated or swollen feeling in the abdominal area and this may possibly be due to a periodic yeast intolerance, i.e. bread, alcohol and other fermented foods may be contributory factors to the recurrence of such problems. In the case of *Candida albicans*, mushrooms, cheese, chocolate or other foods with a high sugar content may exacerbate the problem. The symptoms of swollen and sensitive breasts during this time of the month can be eased greatly by eliminating tobacco, tea, coffee, alcohol, salt, starchy foods, and even saturated fats contained in animal products.

A balanced diet may be a reliable basis for good health, but it is still important for many people to learn to eat less, increase the fibre content in their diet and reduce their intake of sugar, salt, fats and animal proteins. I will provide more detailed information on a specifically devised low-stress diet, as this is highly recommended. It is always beneficial to eat more fruit, vegetables and cereals, particularly rice, and to reduce our intake of sugar and convenience foods.

Just being aware of one's eating habits, particularly during the few days immediately prior to menstruation, will help towards avoiding some of the above problems. Common sense will be necessary if the condition is also related to hypoglycaemia. The patient may have to eat a little more, but should still avoid an excessive intake of carbohydrates. For patients who are subject to depression, it is advisable to eat little and often, and special care must be taken to reduce the intake of coffee, tea and alcohol. The same advice applies for patients who tend to feel more irritable. In cases of unusually severe fluid retention, which is called oedema, the intake of salt must be drastically reduced. Although most of this advice is actually common sense, it is nevertheless necessary during the child-bearing years to be aware of these facts and act accordingly. Good nutrition is a prerequisite for good health.

Some special rules apply for women who suffer from menstrual or premenstrual stress symptoms. The first enemy for such women is sugar. Under no circumstances should the blood sugar level be allowed to fluctuate drastically. As we have learned from the previous chapter, progesterone is produced by the ovaries and is an essential part of the regulating process. If too much progesterone is produced it would cause the adrenaline factor to shoot up. The accumulation of adrenaline, which causes so many problems for women with menstrual symptoms, needs to be carefully controlled, which is why it is important to maintain the blood sugar at a balanced level. To achieve this, unrefined carbohydrates can be of great help. During the time of menstruation it is beneficial to eat brown rice or some other starchy food, as long as it is wholesome and unrefined, e.g. potatoes, rye or oats. It is also advisable to eat relatively small quantities and at frequent intervals. This will also help to avoid bingeing, which is a very common symptom and usually follows craving, which a lot of women experience.

Some women with menstrual symptoms tell me that they feel better for having some chocolate or indulging in an occasional cream cake. This is very often just in the mind, because as the highly refined sugar is absorbed into the bloodstream, it gives the blood sugar level a slight boost. Often patients feel worse afterwards. I must emphasise the importance of eating "good" carbohydrates, which should be unrefined and should be taken in combination with extra vegetable proteins. Additional vitamins, minerals and trace elements will probably also help.

It is important, as I have said, for women who experience menstrual symptoms to eat little and often and it is always a good idea to take some extra starch with you when setting out on a long journey. If the correct foods are taken there is no need to worry about putting on weight; indeed, it should not be used as an excuse for gaining weight. Try taking some extra fruit, remembering that a carrot or an apple can prevent hunger pangs. If you follow this advice you will find it is worth it.

You may be full of good intentions but lacking in motivation. That is the time to remember that in the long run eating a carrot, an apple or a banana, will make you feel a lot better than munching a few biscuits or a bar of chocolate. Just remember how ill you can feel if you experience a periodic allergic reaction, and this would be even more stressful during the time of menstruation. The effects are no less when they have been caused by something that is generally considered as "innocent", such as a biscuit or an extra spoonful of sugar. These cause a rapid rise in the blood sugar level, inevitably followed by an equally sharp drop, leaving you tired, depressed and bad-tempered. The secret, then, lies in a well-balanced diet. It is worth knowing that the sweet potato — the yam — encourages the production of progesterone; for this reason the yam is excellent for those women who suffer from menstrual problems. Because the level of progesterone is exceptionally high during pregnancy, this is one of the reasons described in my book *Living Without Arthritis* why so many pregnant women who normally suffer arthritic pains experience no symptoms at all during pregnancy. Drink plenty of water to cleanse the system and also herbal teas will give a boost during this particular time of the month.

You may have heard the expression, "You are what you eat". Remember that a slight adaptation of this is equally valid: "You are what you drink". Especially in today's society I know how difficult it can be to eat a sensible diet. According to a recently released report, women in the UK admit to eating too much junk food. Many of these foods have lost their nutrients during the manufacturing process. Fortunately, there is a growing interest among women in how they can grow older in good health. Ask yourself if your dietary balance is right. Do you feel lethargic, drained or disorientated during your menstrual period, or do you suffer from mood swings, headaches or abdominal pains? Do you crave sugar, bread, biscuits or alcohol? Do you experience vaginal burning, itching or a discharge? If these symptoms are familiar it could be that you have a problem related to *Candida albicans*.

If you use your common sense, you will realise that it is of little use to have an extra drink in order to forget about these problems. Unfortunately, I have been told this story only too often. Yet alcohol does not represent an escape and only serves to exacerbate existing problems. A woman assimilates alcohol differently to a man, as in women the breakdown of alcohol occurs at a much slower rate. Often, if a woman drinks during the premenstrual period or during ovulation, she will be influenced by alcohol much more quickly than at other times of the month. It upsets me greatly having to diagnose women who should be in their prime as suffering from cirrhosis of the liver or alcohol poisoning. In such cases it is not only the liver that concerns me, since the whole hormonal reproductive system of a woman can become very erratic, and there is also the increased danger of breast cancer. It is always unwise to rely on just another drink in an attempt to fight off depression. Inevitably, the drinker sinks deeper and deeper into the quagmire of depression and requires a second and third drink and before they know where they are, they have come to rely on the bottle. Within a relatively short period of time they have joined the ranks of alcoholics and become more and more negative in their outlook on life. Their relationship with the husband and family inevitably deteriorates and they become isolated from normal life. I will say again that alcohol can never be the answer.

Under these circumstances adopting a balanced diet is essential and the food that is substituted can become really appetising if balanced eating habits are adopted. Unless we eat an appropriate and nutritional diet we will invite many problems, because we rely on food to supply the body with the correct vitamins, minerals and trace elements. A lack of any of these will only aggravate menstrual symptoms. In such a dietary regime it is always preferable to eat organically grown wholefoods, if they can be obtained. I know that this is not always possible and therefore some deficiencies may have to be supplemented with vitamin preparations. The diet should be based on vegetables, fruit, wholegrains and some seafood, the latter being important for maintaining the essential fatty acids balance. Nuts and seeds also contain essential nutrients and together with vegetables and fruit are particularly good sources of nutrition for the hormone-producing organs.

It is not essential to follow a vegetarian diet, but it is well worth knowing that fish is much better than meat for hormone control, as it is a good source of essential fatty acids. If, for some reason, it is too difficult to follow a well-balanced diet, a vitamin supplement may be taken, and in the next chapter I will provide more detailed advice on this aspect. Initially it is probable that a little extra time may be involved in the preparation of a wholesome diet, but it soon becomes a way of life. Remember that investing in our health is the best investment one can possibly make for a healthy future.

During the reproductive stage of life, we realise that our health depends to a large extent on the relationships we had with our parents — from the foetus stage through to infancy. Nowadays much more attention is given to pregnancy, childbirth, breastfeeding and parenting practices, including a move towards longer maternity leave to ensure that the primal needs which are essential for laying a good foundation to the immune system can be met.

The consumption of food grown in poor soil, under poor conditions or with the aid of artificial fertilisers, deprives us of the opportunity to absorb the necessary minerals from our daily food intake, resulting in trace element deficiencies. Minerals are important for our health and they are totally absent from white sugar and refined, cooked or baked flour products. A lack of minerals causes the body to release glucose into the bloodstream far too quickly. The sudden increase of glucose in the bloodstream in turn causes the liver and pancreas to be confronted with a state of emergency. The liver is burdened with the task of converting glucose into glycogen and the refined sugar and flour products, which only provide empty calories, put the pancreas and liver under stress. This process all happens very quickly.

Surveys have shown that one person in four needs extra vitamins and minerals. As a naturopath it is my belief that if the diet is correctly balanced, there should be no need for supplements. Unfortunately, this principle is practically impossible to maintain nowadays as our food is being adulterated with preservatives, flavourings, colourings and artificial fertilisers. As a result it lacks the required vitamins, minerals and trace elements — and in the case of women prone to menstrual and premenstrual tension these deficiencies become much more pronounced. I will say more on this topic in a later chapter.

The World Health Organisation has launched a

campaign to educate people on the need for a healthy balance in food. It is widely accepted that in modern food-processing procedures many chemical additives are considered essential, with the result that there is very little vital force left in processed food. Nutritional research must be directed towards educating people in the importance of a balanced diet.

Many of my patients who once suffered from menstrual and premenstrual tension and who changed their diet as part of their treatment, have spoken with surprise of the far-reaching effects of what may have been only a minor dietary adjustment. With remarkable regularity I receive letters from patients who have previously consulted me on the subject of menstrual symptoms. They mostly write to let me know how grateful they are for the reversal in their condition after changing their diet. Basically, it is relatively simple to take the first steps towards better nutritional management. Always keep your sugar intake as low as possible. Start eating extra fruit and vegetables. If you are feeling a bit low and the craving for something sweet becomes irresistible, try taking some honey. Be sparing with salt, tea, coffee and alcohol, and reduce your intake of dairy produce and animal fats. I can assure you that by following such simple advice you will progress a long way towards overcoming this tension and stress. Should there be any *Candida albicans* problems, thrush, or cystitis, further dietary advice follows later.

Dietary requirements vary so widely that the best diet for an individual is generally one which has been tailor-made to suit. However, many years ago Dr Alfred Vogel and I designed some guidelines for what can best be described as a low-stress diet.

This diet may be adapted to suit individual needs and serves merely as a set of general guidelines. According to the patient's condition and circumstances, it may be complemented by supplementary vitamins, minerals and trace elements.

Low-stress diet
Breakfast
Muesli mixed with juice of an orange, a grated apple, half a banana or other fruit. One or two pieces of rye crispbread or wholemeal bread spread with natural vegetable margarine (sunflower or corn oil). One cup of tea after the meal, preferably peppermint, rosehip or chamomile. "Bambu" coffee from the Bioforce range may be used as an alternative.

Midday meal
A plate of fresh vegetables, especially carrots and beetroot. Use other raw and cooked vegetables when in season. The fresh vegetables can be mixed with a dressing made from olive or sunflower oil with a little lemon juice or celery juice. Baked or steamed potatoes in their jackets may be eaten with the vegetables.
For dessert take yoghurt (low fat) with honey.

Evening meal
Muesli, then fresh fruit salad. If indigestion is a problem, do not eat these together. Vegetable soup made from vegetable leftovers, with the possible addition of apples, radishes, figs, leeks and tomatoes, flavoured with Kelpamare seasoning.
Use salt sparingly, and remember that a little Herbamare salt is much better for your health. (NB Kelpamare and Herbamare are both products available in the Bioforce range.)

General advice
Animal fat is prohibited. Use eggs sparingly. No white flour or white sugar (or products made with them), pork, sausages, bacon or ham. Cut down or, even better, omit

completely, coffee, alcohol, nicotine and sweets. Try to take some daily exercise outdoors in order to obtain some fresh air. Increased physical activity is recommended; for example, try walking to the shops or work instead of driving.

5

Supplements

IN THE PREVIOUS CHAPTER I pointed out that a balanced diet should supply the body with all the nutrients which it requires for optimum health. Yet we must realise that because of modern food processing, cooking methods and our lifestyle, much of the nutritional value disappears from our food before we eat it and many people certainly need some extra supplements. During the menstrual and premenstrual period women's nutritional needs change almost daily and therefore this is an important area to investigate when trying to reduce menstrual symptoms.

I have been trained in the old-fashioned naturopathic ways and I wish that it was still possible to treat people according to my forebears' principles, i.e. with pure food, water and air. Unfortunately, this is out of the question today because of environmental changes. When we consider the way our basic foods are encouraged to grow in poor soil conditions, with the aid of artificial fertilisers, the pre-processing, the additives, and the water we drink, we cannot fail to realise that nutritional standards are slipping. When we take all these factors into account we must be sensible and look carefully for ways to redress the balance. Fortunately, extra help can be obtained in the form of vitamin and mineral supplements.

Generally speaking, in most European countries little attention is given to this subject, whereas more comprehensive studies have taken place in the United States and Canada, from where I have gathered much information. There the alarm has been raised and the need for nutritional supplements has been recognised, possibly because of the methods of food processing, fast food and junk food habits which are more prevalent there. When pollution and its effects are added to these factors we cannot fail to realise the risks to the quality of our nutrition and the need to learn about supplementary nutrition.

Three essential requirements for combating menstrual and premenstrual tension are vitamin B_6, magnesium and evening primrose oil. Unfortunately, it does not stop there; our overall approach must be revised as we know that many other minerals and trace elements can be deficient. Our body is not capable of storing or utilising each and every vitamin if the assimilating minerals are lacking. In the United Kingdom selenium and zinc — both vital minerals — are in extremely short supply in our diets. When certain vitamins, minerals and trace elements are not readily available, I often hear my female patients reel off lists of complaints such as headaches, water retention, weight gain and depression. All of these are listed as the more common symptoms of the premenstrual syndrome.

Calcium, for instance, is the most abundant mineral in the body and most of it is found in our bones, but a small amount of calcium is found outside the bones, where it functions in a number of essential ways. Millions of women who suffer from menstrual symptoms are found to be lacking vitamins and minerals as a result of dieting for weight reduction or because they take the contraceptive pill, and in the case of calcium deficiency there is a greater risk of developing osteoporosis later on in life. We must understand the task of our skeleton. This framework of our body is alive and must remain active. If it should refuse to act, the muscles and ligaments of our body would become dormant and atrophic and we would lose control of them. Other factors to consider are the nerves, which carry impulses, and the veins, which carry nutrients to the bones. We also have blood circulation in the marrow of each bone.

The next consideration is the cartilage. At each joint where the bones meet we find cartilage separating one from the other. This cartilage acts as a cushion between the joints. The cartilage receives lubrication from the bone marrow. We must keep our skeleton erect in order to maintain the proper lubrication in each joint. It is the lubrication that causes our joints to be flexible. If power in our bones is lacking, this is caused by a shortage of calcium. Calcium builds the foundation. Phosphate and calcium react together to calcify or harden the bone. Protein prevents the bone from breaking when tension is applied. If we experience pain in the bones of our hands, it shows a lack of calcium. If the bone is hard and brittle there is a lack of silica.

Our bones are composed of various minerals (69 per cent), organic substances, moisture and water. This analysis can be broken down as follows:

organic substances — 31 per cent
calcium phosphate — 58.2 per cent
calcium carbonate — 7 per cent

calcium fluoride — 1.5 per cent
magnesium phosphate — 1.3 per cent
sodium chloride — 1.0 per cent

In this analysis there is no mention of sulphur or silica, but there is a large proportion of calcium in different combinations. We know that the largest percentage of calcium in the body is to be found in our bones and teeth. However, it is also essential in the process of blood-clotting and muscle contraction. Calcium levels in the body are dependent on several factors, and deficiencies are usually caused by a lack of vitamin D or by taking steroid drugs or the contraceptive pill. In the case of the latter, there are advantages and disadvantages with this method of birth control.

In 1960, when the contraceptive pill first became available, it seemed to be the answer to many people's prayers. However, as with many new "wonder drugs", it has failed to live up to its original promise. Despite clinical trials, it seems that the testing was insufficient and now, thirty years on, it has become clear that the oestrogen content of the pill can be reduced by half and still be as effective in the prevention of conception.

As far as the advantages of the contraceptive pill are concerned, it does help to regulate an unpredictable monthly cycle. It also helps to eliminate the pain and discomfort sometimes caused by menstruation, and prevents anaemia. It is also thought to reduce the risk of ovarian cysts or ovarian cancer. However the pill also has some disadvantages, one of which is the danger of osteoporosis. The pill still ought to be considered as a very potent medication, as it affects every system in the body. It has not yet been completely investigated and it remains possible that long-term use of this method of birth control could have carcinogenic effects, particularly with regard to the cervix and breast. If you are concerned about this risk, remember that there are other methods of birth control that can be considered to achieve the same effect more safely.

A report on the findings of an investigation carried out by "Ladycare" states that 62 per cent of the women interviewed between the age of 18 and 24 were taking the contraceptive pill. This figure fell to 21 per cent for the age group 25–39, and was as low as 6 per cent for those aged 40–49 and 1 per cent for the 50-plus age group. Among those interviewed there did not appear to be much concern about a possible relationship between taking the pill and developing thrombosis, cancer or heart disease. Yet for those women who do use the contraceptive pill, some supplementary vitamins, minerals and trace elements are important, most especially calcium.

In my experience one of the best calcium preparations available is Urticalcin, a product from the Bioforce range. This is an excellent homoeopathic combination of calcium and silicium, which should be prescribed if a calcium deficiency is suspected. It is ideally suited for the purpose of building bones, combating brittle nails and hair loss. Its use is recommended for menstrual or premenstrual tension and during pregnancy. It also acts as a neutraliser for excessive amounts of acid in the body.

A deficiency of the mineral magnesium is also often a major factor in menstrual and premenstrual tension. This link has been confirmed as the result of many clinical trials, and studies have shown the effect of magnesium deficiency in relation to other menstrual symptoms. An excellent remedy, containing the essentials for treating menstrual or premenstrual tension is a Nature's Best product called Optivite, available in the Lamberts' range. Optivite is a multi-vitamin preparation designed especially for menstruating women and to which all the essential minerals and trace elements have been added to a hypo-allergic base.

I have worked with Optivite for some time now and many of my female patients have reported that they were delighted with the tremendous improvement in their menstrual symptoms achieved with the help of this product.

Dr Guy Abraham, former professor of obstetrics and gynaecology at the UCLA School of Medicine, turned to nutritional supplementation after years of research into hormones and how their production is affected by vitamins and minerals. He found that many women were at risk in this respect through not obtaining sufficient nutrients from their diet and that the dietary habits of others were depleting the nutritional value of their food. Optivite is the end result of his quest for a multivitamin and mineral supplement that would cover the most common areas of shortfall. The most effective combination of nutrients was selected after clinical trials in America showed that some ingredients needed to be present in precise proportions or they could not be fully absorbed. Dr Abraham believes that Optivite is the only women's supplement that has passed bio-availability studies.

Increasing numbers of British women are taking Optivite following trials arranged by the Women's Nutritional Advisory Service, which has emphasised that Optivite works best as part of a complete health-building programme that includes adequate exercise, a proper diet and sufficient rest and relaxation. It is recommended that 1–3 tablets are taken twice daily with meals, preferably breakfast and lunch.

The medical profession is now coming round to recognising the power of diet to influence health, both positively and negatively, and since 1984 the Women's Nutritional Advisory Service has worked very hard to relieve the unhappiness that is being caused by menstrual and premenstrual tension.

MENSTRUAL AND PREMENSTRUAL TENSION

From an article in the journal *Drug Intelligence and Clinical Pharmacology* of October 1985, I quote:

Another nutritional etiologic theory of PMT surrounds the role of Vitamin B_6, or its active co-enzyme form, pyridoxinal phosphate, in oestrogen metabolism and in the synthesis of tryptophan and dopamine. Vitamin B_6 was proposed in the 1940s to be related to menstrual symptoms when it was observed that pyridoxine deficiency in rats seemed to impair the oestrogen metabolism. It was speculated that a similar deficiency in humans might lead to the apparent oestrogen excess seen in PMT. However, normal oestrogen metabolism has been documented in women with severe pyridoxine deficiency. More recently it has been documented that Vitamin B_6 is involved as a co-enzyme in the final step of biosynthesis of dopamine and serotonin. Conversion reactions of L-tryptophan to seratonin and to kynurenine metabolites are catalysed by pyridoxinal phosphate and tryptophan pyrrolase, respectively. It has been proposed that oestrogen excess, such as that resulting from oral contraceptive use, increases the requirements for pyridoxinal phosphate. It is possible that a relative deficiency of pyridoxinal phosphate occurs, leading to a reduction in the synthesis of serotonin. It is a widespread belief that reduced serotonin is associated with symptoms seen both in patients with PMT and those who use oral contraceptives. Finally, it has been suggested that a deficiency of Vitamin B_6 could result in decreased dopamine synthesis, leading to prolactin excess and mastalgia, another common premenstrual problem.

From this article the scientific evidence for the crucial role of vitamin B_6 appears very clear-cut and this has been taken into consideration in the Optivite formula.

It is quite a few years now since I first introduced oil of evening primrose to my practice in Scotland. The seeds of this attractive yellow flower have been a great blessing and have enabled me to help many women to overcome their menstrual and premenstrual symptoms. The nutrients known as essential fatty acids (EFA) are necessary dietary factors for two main reasons: firstly they are needed for the functioning of the cell membranes in the tissues of the body, and secondly they work as precursors of highly reactive, short-lived molecules known as prostaglandins.

I have already touched upon the influence of prostaglandins, and we also know that it is the prostaglandin E1 that controls the menstrual cycle. Gammalinolenic acid (GLA), which is dependent on linoleic acid in the diet, is also essential. Oil of evening primrose comprises 9 per cent GLA and 70 per cent linoleic acid and clinical studies have proved this natural product to be of immense value in alleviating menstrual symptoms.

At St Thomas' Hospital Medical School a study was performed on sixty-eight women who all suffered from severe menstrual symptoms. Following treatment with oil of evening primrose: 66 per cent had a complete remission of all symptoms and a further 22 per cent claimed a partial improvement. Moreover, twenty-six of the thirty-six women with cyclical breast pain experienced complete relief and a further five, partial relief.

Recently, double-blind cross-over trials using oil of evening primrose with women suffering from menstrually related irritable bowel syndrome showed significant results. Of the thirty-six women who completed the trial, four were withdrawn and two did not comply with the study. Only seventeen women reported no change in their symptoms. An improvement during one phase of the trial was reported by nineteen women, and when the double-blind code was broken all nineteen were found to have improved whilst taking oil of evening primrose, with none reporting improvement while on placebos. This again was reassuring, and several new oil of evening primrose preparations of different composition have also produced good results.

In my book *Traditional Home and Herbal Remedies* more detailed information can be found on the effects of oil of evening primrose.

As nutrients, essential fatty acids are just as important as vitamins and minerals. They cannot be manufactured by the body and so have to be supplied by our diet. They are not only integral components of cell walls, but are metabolised to form chemical messengers known as prostaglandins, hormone-like substances which control many different metabolic pathways. One of the most important of these messengers, prostaglandin E1 (PGE1), controls several body functions, including blood pressure regulation and cholesterol production.

Essential fatty acids are all unsaturated, but before they can be metabolised to form prostaglandins they have to be converted to even more unsaturated fatty acids such as gammalinolenic acid (GLA), a precursor of PGE1. This process may sometimes be inefficient and therefore a dietary source of GLA can be useful.

Human breast milk is one of the best-known suppliers of correctly balanced EFA and GLA, and experts have tried for many years to find a more convenient source. The evening primrose plant is one of the richest natural sources of GLA, from which the body produces many of the vital prostaglandins, and its oil has now become the standard EFA and GLA supplement. Nature's Best primrose oil, for example, is encapsulated with gelatin, glycerin and purified water.

If we look at all the groups of supplements, Optivite, oil of evening primrose and Urticalcin would form as good a base as possible to combat painful periods. For the PMT-A anxiety, the PMT-H hydration group, the PMT-C craving group, or the PMT-D depression group other specific remedies may be needed, which I will deal with in the next chapter.

Dr Guy Abraham, as well as formulating the excellent supplement Optivite, has unravelled the menstrual symptoms in these particular groups. He has done an excellent job and found that each group experiences different symptoms. However, an inadequate diet seems to be common to them all, and of course stress and emotional factors.

Taking a few positive steps such as those I have described may bring about the same reaction as expressed by one of my patients whose menstrual symptoms had become a thing of the past. She wrote of her gratitude and new-found zest for life in a letter from which I quote: "Life has become wonderful again. I am now in harmony again with myself and nature, as you promised me."

6

Homoeopathic and Herbal Medicine

BEARING IN MIND the different categories of menstrual or premenstrual tension, it is important to advise a standard treatment method. Every individual is different. If the menstrual symptoms of a hundred women were to be listed, we would find that the details of each would vary slightly. This is yet another reason why homoeopathy and herbal medicine play such a tremendous role, as these forms of medicine allow us to look for safe alternatives to re-establish harmony in our bodies.

Let us look first at what homoeopathy has to offer. Many books have been written on this subject, by advocates and opponents alike. Instead of going into great detail and lengthy explanations, I would simply like to point out that this medical science is founded upon the basic principle established by Paracelsus: *"similis similibus curentur"* — like cures like. Samuel Hahnemann was the founder of homoeopathy as we know it today and he formulated the fundamental basics of his medical beliefs in such a way that homoeopathy has been allowed to develop into a completely separate and self-sufficient form of medical treatment.

It all started with a slow but steadily growing dissatisfaction with the current medicine of his time, and with the severe action of allopathic drugs. Consequently, Hahnemann decided to examine the effects of homoeopathic extracts on perfectly healthy people. He tried the plant *Cinchona* (a cure for malaria) on himself and was amazed to discover that it produced in him the very symptoms of the disease for which it was prescribed. He repeated this experiment using different extracts on other volunteers and his findings and interpretations eventually led to the foundation of homoeopathy as we know it today. By prescribing a drug that produced artificial symptoms in a healthy person — the same as those suffered by a patient — the body's own defence mechanism was stimulated.

Remedies diluted one part in one hundred more than thirty times over became commonplace in homoeopathic prescribing, which led to ridicule from allopathic doctors and conventional scientists, who claimed that none of the original substance could possibly remain. Yet, as I have mentioned in some of the earlier chapters of this book, it only requires a minor vibration to cause a change in the situation, and remembering this may help us to understand that even the lowest potency in homoeopathy could alter some unwanted characteristics. I must admit that the body's reaction still amazes me occasionally, even after thirty-five years in practice. As a natural holistic alternative, homoeopathic medicine is completely safe and does not produce uncomfortable or debilitating side-effects.

Homoeopathy is based on natural substances and with regard to menstrual symptoms homoeopathy takes into consideration the emotional, mental and physical aspects required to restore the body's natural balance. There is very little new under the sun despite our modern knowledge; it was back in the fourth century BC when Hippocrates — the Father of Medicine — taught that our food is our medicine and our medicine our food.

The abundance of natural sources — animal, vegetable, mineral, biological and herbal — from which homoeopathic medicines are derived, is infinite and therefore allows practitioners numerous options from which to choose the right remedies and/or combinations. Einstein must have understood some of the fundamental principles of homoeopathy and he applied aspects of them in his own specific theories. He said that a field of energy was the only reality and that the material which came from space is extremely intense in this field. In any criticism on low potencies, this shows us again that dynamic potential dilution actually increases the potential effect on this great field of energy, which is the body. It is surprising how quickly negative energy can be changed. This becomes apparent when we see an arthritic condition develop because of a hormonal imbalance in a young woman. When we give her the remedy *Rhus Tox* — poison ivy — the smallest possible amount will produce a reaction, which appears to exacerbate the symptoms, as before.

"Like cures like." This homoeopathic philosophy never ceases to amaze. How surprising that even the lowest potency can effect a change in one's condition. Take for instance a patient who suffers from menorrhagia or a heavy menstrual flow. In such a case I may decide to prescribe a product called Sepia, which does a marvellous job in regulating the flow. If I were to explain that Sepia is a by-product of the cuttlefish, people may wonder why I prescribe this for excessive perspiration, or heavy menstrual flow, or vaginal discharge. Yet it has proved to be of great value in controlling the above-mentioned conditions.

If, however, the menstrual flow is quite slight, the ovaries may require extra cleansing. A homoeopathic dose is used, which takes effect within a few days, and also results in more regular periods. I usually combine the use of this remedy with Kelpasan, which is a product obtained from marine algae found deep in the Pacific Ocean. When taken together these remedies will encourage a normal menstrual flow and regulate the menstrual cycle.

For women who suffer from amenorrhoea, which is an absence of menstruation, I advise the use of Ovarium D3. Many women can vouch for the efficacy of combining Kelpasan and Ovarium, as well as taking mustard seed baths. This combination has also proved extremely effective in the treatment of young women with anorexia nervosa, which causes severe disturbances in the menstrual cycle.

When excessive pain, or dysmenorrhoea, is experienced during menstruation, whether it takes the form of cramps, lower backache, dizziness or headaches, Belladonna D4 can often provide speedy relief from the symptoms. Although this lovely plant with its beautiful flowers is highly poisonous, when prescribed in a homoeopathic potency it is an effective form of treatment for the pain caused by menstrual cramps.

One of the most useful combinations for general menstrual symptoms in my experience is Optivite together with Dr Vogel's Menstruation Formula (available in the Bioforce range). This combination is recommended for amenorrhoea, an insufficient or excessive menstrual flow, painful menstruation and also if the patient suffers from a whitish vaginal discharge. Menstruation Formula in particular has a normalising effect on the menstrual cycle.

Looking at the bounty of nature, we will see that it gives us an endless supply of possible combinations for herbal remedies: countless flowers, leaves, roots and even tree barks. When we examine further the wealth of detail available from natural sources we can begin to appreciate Dr Bach's reasoning. Dr Bach worked at his remedies and combinations fired by the conviction that plants, roots or leaves hold the key to many health problems.

It is my belief too that nature supplies us with the means for finding a cure to our health problems and not simply with the materials for the manufacture of drugs. Natural products should remain natural so that they can fit into a holistic treatment pattern. Extracting or crystallising this wonderful living material into different components will only create yet another drug and although herbal medicine may be a benign form of allopathy, the facts remain that its remedies come from an entirely natural origin. In the practice of herbal medicine the diagnosis and treatment relates to the individual, rather than to a named disease. Allopathic treatment may involve the prescription of a single drug for the treatment of a specific condition, but herbal treatment will work mildly and gently to rebalance the entire body, ensuring that there are no toxic side-effects.

This wonderful vital force that lives in everyone aspires to life and is chiefly concerned with maintaining its equilibrium. Herbalism too treats the patient, not the disease, by directing the vital force and encouraging it with herbal remedies which stimulate the body's own defences to produce the desired return to positive health.

As a result of my frequent radio talks I have received hundreds of letters regarding menstrual and premenstrual tension. Many listeners obtain relief by using one of the lesser known medicinal herbs — sage. Isn't it amazing that what is generally regarded as a culinary herb has such a tremendous power? If it had not been researched we would never have known that it contains a high content of potassium, calcium, silicium and zinc, which are carried right into the brain tissue. Sage has a direct effect on the pituitary gland, which in turn goes on to influence the entire hormonal system.

I am pleased to see that an increasing number of Chinese remedies are now being accepted in our Western culture. These herbal remedies have been used and tested for many centuries in China, and now there is a grudging admiration for them elsewhere. During my own studies in China I was often astounded by their usefulness and effectiveness.

For patients who like to mix their own herbs, the following recipe is an excellent remedy for painful menstruation and for menstrual disorders in general, as it is designed to tone, regulate and strengthen the whole reproductive system. Mix together the following ingredients:

1 part raspberry — which relaxes the pelvic muscles;
3 parts golden seal — for dysmenorrhoea;
1 part false unicorn — a stimulative tonic for the ovaries;
1 part ginger — an excellent menstruation suppressor;
1 part cramp bark — an anti-spasmodic and sedative;
1 part uva-ursi — for excessive menstruation;
1 part cayenne — a good general stimulant;
1 part blessed thistle.

I discovered the instructions for this old herbal combination remedy at Napier's Herbal Dispensary. The combined dried herbs can be used as a blend for herbal tea. One cup of the herbal infusion should be drunk morning and evening.

While on the subject of drinks, I must stress that women who suffer from menstrual disorders should aim to reduce their consumption of coffee, tea and alcohol, which are all stimulants, particularly during menstruation. Nowadays there are a number of very pleasant alternatives, such as Bioforce Bambu coffee, or herbal teas. There is an extremely wide choice of such teas, which are easily obtained from health food stores, but I would especially recommend peppermint, rosehip or any of the fruit teas.

I have been pleased to see the renewed interest in herbal teas, which are basically much healthier than ordinary tea, and in this context I must tell you about the Herbal Health Tea, the recipe for which was compiled by my grandmother many years ago. This tea is now widely used and as well as being a refreshing drink, it has a positive influence on our health.

All over the world the interest in herbal medicine is growing fast. This should not be surprising when we consider that man has instinctively, since his creation, used herbal preparations to alleviate many cases of suffering. Why use chemical ingredients such as aspirin, if the same result can be achieved by taking a natural remedy such as Petadolor? The main ingredient of this herbal remedy is butterbur extract and it acts as a calming and relaxing agent against pains caused by cramps, such as migraine, menstrual discomfort, and neck and back pains. A few tablets daily will alleviate such problems as effectively as any chemical painkiller.

I was surprised to learn, on my travels to China and India, that Chinese herbalism and the Ayurveda herbalism practised in India are commonly used in conjunction with orthodox medicine. In the Far East herbal teas and drinks are now widely accepted as a form of medical treatment because they provide a natural way to restore harmony within the body.

Another problem that is often experienced during the menstrual cycle is a lack of bladder control. This can be easily solved with the help of hot or cold water sitz baths, and in my book *Water — Healer or Poison?* I provide plenty of examples of these and other water treatment methods. Never ignore such symptoms and remember to drink plenty of water — barley water is helpful and so are mineral waters. Keep warm with hot-water bottles, and avoid sweet foods, alcohol and spices. An inflammation of the bladder lining can lead to uncomfortable or burning sensations when passing urine, and a pressing need to empty the bladder very frequently. These symptoms can also be a sign of cystitis or a bacterial or viral infection. The lower abdomen is particularly vulnerable to infection during menstruation. If, however, it is only a bladder problem then the remedy Cystoforce will be ideal. Cystoforce is a fresh herb preparation that can be used to treat a whole range of bladder problems, such as a general weakness of the bladder, cystitis or bedwetting, without the risk of side-effects.

Try to ensure that there is no yeast infection as this could lead to thrush, which is a vaginal infection that causes a thick white discharge and intense local irritation. Thrush can be caused by a yeast infection like *Monilia* or *Candida albicans* and help should always be sought from a qualified practitioner, as this problem can quickly get out of hand. Do not forget that the female hormone progesterone inhibits the formation of the protective lining of the bladder, while the hormone oestrogen increases it. Although such problems are more likely to arise during the menopause, they can arise at other times. Although there is as yet no concrete evidence, research points to a possible link between the use of the contraceptive pill and the incidence of bladder and bacterial infections.

Thrush is by no means exclusive to women undergoing the menopause and it is quite common for women who have not yet reached the end of their reproductive stage of life to experience vaginal complaints and thrush. Always ensure that the necessary steps are taken to overcome this tiresome irritation and you will be spared much future discomfort.

7

Cranial Osteopathy

WHAT IS THE connection between premenstrual tension and the skull and cranium? In previous chapters we have read how the master glands — the composer and the conductor — are safely tucked away within our skulls. By the application of light pressure or touch these highly sensitive glands can be influenced, either positively or negatively, but it is vitally important that this is only done by professionally trained practitioners who possess an in-depth knowledge of the subject. Before providing you with a more detailed explanation of cranial osteopathy, I will tell you a little more about the skull and the bones, which will make the whole process easier to understand.

It is possible for the bones of the skull to become slightly displaced and this can be caused by any one of a variety of reasons. Let us first look at the jawbone. If the left side of the skull is low, the right side is forced to rise out of its usual position. This causes the teeth on the left side of the mouth to close much more firmly than those on the right side, with the result that we will be inclined to chew our food on the left side of the mouth. By doing so, we take the pressure off the teeth on the right side which will stop the nerve action and circulation of the blood to both the upper and lower teeth on that side of the face. In many cases this can lead to toothache, a dislocated jaw or, what is worse, problems affecting the temporo-mandibular (TM) joint, and I have treated many patients with premenstrual syndrome for this last complaint.

If the lower jawbone has dropped, this can cause the sinus and facial bones to become twisted out of alignment. By standing in front of a mirror and placing one finger of the right hand under the right cheekbone and one finger of the left hand under the left cheekbone, we can tell just how much the facial bones have moved out of position. Such unnatural pressure on the facial bones will cause problems with the antria, which are cavities in the sinus, as well as with the adenoids, possibly resulting in a blockage of the sinuses.

On close examination of the facial bone structure one eye will often appear to be lower than the other. This is the result of the facial bones being out of position or alignment. Then the frontal or forehead bone will show the same signs, thus moving the bone of the forehead down on the left side, causing the left eye to be lower. As the left side of the frontal part of the skull moves downwards, it automatically causes the back of the skull on the same side to move upwards. This will interfere with the position of the mastoid gland, causing unnatural pressure on the medulla and interfering with the person's sight and hearing. It causes the mastoid bone to rise, corresponding with the back of the skull. This movement will, in turn, prevent the head from being aligned correctly on the atlas, which is the topmost bone of the spine, impinging on the nerves and throat. This can result in the circulation being impeded to different parts of the head and face and increase the likelihood of stumbling, falling or turning an ankle. This can be noticed in people who suffer from intermittent staggering, or who are afraid of heights. This can also be noticed when climbing a ladder, or looking down from high buildings, where patients may suffer from dizziness or vertigo.

The causes for such problems are located in the brain, directly under the temporal bone which is just above the ear. The left side of the forehead being lower than it should be exerts pressure upon this bone, in turn causing pressure on the brain. The corresponding bone on the opposite side of the head will protrude. All this brings pressure to bear on the centre of balance in the brain. This pressure not only causes the problems described above, but also unbalances the entire thinking process, the individual willpower and the action of the entire body.

If the skull is higher on one side than the other, it will cause pressure on the brain, preventing the function of the relevant portion of the brain and the nervous system that connects with vital parts of our body. The skull moving out of position or alignment in this way could easily lead to the appearance of lymphatic tumours in the skull. Such movements only have to be infinitesimal to cause far-reaching problems.

If the forehead is out of alignment — one side higher than the other — this will be obvious in the bone structure above the eyes. If there is a depression in the skull just above the forehead, the neck will become stiff, the shoulders will move out of alignment and problems will be experienced in the hands and wrists.

On either side of the top centre of the skull there is a direct connection between the underlying portion of the brain and the feet, especially the toes and metatarsal arches. If a defect arises in the back of the skull, we may experience trouble with both eyes and ears. These misplaced bones of the skull cause pressure on the brain or the cells of the brain connected with different parts of our body. There is also an opening in the top of our skull through which we make contact with the conscious system. Think about the misplaced sections of the skull and the great influence and pressure that is exerted on the nerves and the circulation of the head and face, and the pressure that is brought to bear on the different sections of the brain. It may take several manipulative treatments to return the skull to its correct position, thereby relieving the nerves and the blood circulation.

One simple method for women who suffer from menstrual or premenstrual tension is to press gently with both thumbs above the tops of the ears. Just above the ears there are two small indentations and by gently rubbing both thumbs upwards and downwards, a good deal of pressure will be relieved. The advice given in this chapter may appear too simple to be effective, but a positive attitude will achieve positive results; positive action will lead to improved mentality and a change in the conscious system.

Our first consideration always should be the skull and its elastic fibre. Next we should look for ways of restoring the function of the neck, shoulders and arms, which results in greater suppleness of the whole spine. All this can be done by manipulation of the skull. More often than not if we have a crooked skeleton, we will find that the problems originate in the skull or cranium. When initially examining patients I often ask the same questions: did they know if their birth had followed a natural pattern or was it a forceps delivery? Was it a difficult birth or a straightforward delivery? Such information helps me to determine whether the skull has suffered as a result of excessive force or pressure. I often advise mothers whose babies have been delivered under difficult conditions that any minor damage to the skull should be looked at by a cranial osteopath. Each part of the body should be able to work freely, which enables the conscious mind to perform without interference and it is for this reason that it is important that cranial osteopathy be considered as an option.

One of my tutors, Dr Denis Brookes, always said that with some simple movements a well-qualified cranial osteopath is capable of changing things that otherwise are likely to cause problems that could last a lifetime. One of his favourite expressions was "Find it, fix it and leave it". This shows how professional he was.

Since 1936 there has been slow progress in the science of endocrinology, and a limited recognition of the belief that our thought processes can influence the endocrine system and therefore our immune system. This is only the beginning. As yet these principles have not been fully explored by endocrinologists and it is now time that the Hahnemann principle should be applied, i.e. that the symptoms should be regarded holistically and the mind, body and soul treated as a whole. We must accept the value of direct stimulation of the endocrine system through the pituitary gland. The metabolic process is improved with tissue nutrition. Gentle absorption of calcium and the ability of the cranial osteopath will bring about great improvement in the treatment of premenstrual tension.

I will now return to my earlier statement that cranial osteopathy is important because the pineal gland and the pituitary gland are tucked away inside the skull. Any cranial misalignment will affect these glands and I will therefore reiterate that it is possible for some problems to originate either accidentally or even during the process of giving birth.

In the ageing process the pituitary gland is greatly influenced by the hypothalamus. If the hypothalamus centres are under pressure, this could be caused by a neck disalignment and a simple adjustment could solve the problem. I may call the pituitary gland the conductor, but it is still part of the chain of seven endocrine glands, where it is strongly influenced by the hypothalamus. Whilst experiencing menstrual symptoms such as fluid retention, blood pressure or possibly depression, it is important to realise that these problems usually arise when the hypothalamus is not being influenced correctly. The application of mild pressure with both hands on the fourth ventricle may lead to some improvement in this particular system. Balance or harmony — whatever we call it — is one of the most important aspects of cranial osteopathic treatment. It may be considered simple, but this treatment in fact involves a complicated study of the way the body works.

It is possible to relieve tension in the cranium by simple hand movements. One of the best methods, and one that can be done by anyone, is to place the left hand on the forehead and the right hand on the neck immediately below the occiput. In my book *Body Energy* I have described many hand movements which can be safely used on the skull by individuals without specialised knowledge.

Many of these methods have proved to be of great help for the relief of menstrual disorders.

Sometimes there may be doubt about the possibility of correcting the damage done by a fractured skull. Whatever the injury, there is always something that can be done and there are always compensations. It will always be worthwhile seeking professional advice. A short while ago I was visited by a lady whose skull had previously been fractured in a traffic accident. She told me how much better she felt since I had instructed her on some self-help methods, which were indeed simple enough for a lay person to follow. Much of the manipulation was administered by her own hands. We managed to sort her problems out and it is useful to know that some of these methods can be applied to a wide range of problems, going beyond menstrual symptoms.

The other day I was asked to examine a baby and my diagnosis was a case of occipual condylitis. There was a displacement in the cranium and with some manipulation the condition was corrected, thus ensuring a better chance for the baby's future. Such injuries to infants at birth are often dismissed, as it is generally thought that in time they will right themselves. This is an assumption we should never make, because if too much time is allowed to lapse, it may no longer be possible to correct the effects of such an injury.

A lady with very severe menstrual symptoms came back to see me recently. Her gratitude was overwhelming and she had been wondering how I had located the source of her problems to a dislocation of the jaw. It had not taken me long to diagnose that the dislocated jaw was the cause of quite severe pressure on the skull. I explained that since the misalignment had been corrected the hormone imbalance would find its own level and she confirmed a tremendous improvement in the problems previously associated with her menstrual cycle.

Yet another patient I treated was found to have problems with the hyoid — a horseshoe-like bone which is ancillary to the cranial system, with many ligaments and muscles attached. Misalignment of the hyoid causes excessive pressure in other parts of the skull.

A further important factor with regard to cranial osteopathy is that it encourages secretions from the endocrine glands into the bloodstream. These are very potent and essential to the body, as they control the nutrition we receive from our food. Our entire physical life is regulated by these important glands and centres. This becomes clear when we consider that the pineal gland affects the liver, the pituitary gland relates to the spleen, the thyroid is linked to the suprarenal and the parathyroid influences the duodenum. As for the reproductive glands, the thymus is linked with the ovaries and the mammaries in females, while in males it influences the prostate, the stomach and the gonads. All this shows what an important role these underrated glands making up the endocrine system have to perform.

Nowadays one of the major causes of disease is tension and emotional stress. We should therefore try and understand what causes the neuro-endocrine functions to be adversely affected. An average person's body contains 62,000 miles of blood vessels all interlaced with nerve fibres, into which adrenaline is released under acute and chronic stress conditions. This can produce a shock syndrome which in some instances can be the cause of long-term problems. Fortunately, such problems can be clinically identified and eradicated with certain treatment methods.

From the outset I had intended to include a few tips on how to use the hands in case of pancreas problems. Place the left hand over the sixth dorsal, cover it with the right hand and maintain this position for some time. If a problem is linked to the adrenals, cover dorsal nine in the same way. For the ovaries it is dorsal number three, which will also help the pituitary and thyroid glands. These are just a few simple tips to remember should a little extra help be required. More detailed information on this subject can be found in my book, *Body Energy*.

The cerebrospinal fluid is one of the most important constituents of the human body. Never forget that each contact on the cranium is a vital spot from which to influence specified areas of the body with precision. When feeling tense and a tranquillising effect is required, encircle the occiput with the palm of the right hand. The occiput is the protruding part of the skull just under the cranium. Place the index finger of the left hand on the centre of the forehead in line with the nose. Never forget that the surface area of the skull has potent reflexes to areas or organs, some of which are bilateral and some are unilateral. Even light pressure, or gentle holding or massaging, can provide great relief. Use the hands in the correct way. Ancient civilisation taught that the positive power is located in the right hand, while the left hand contains negative power. This remains the same whether one is male or female, or right- or left-handed. The intelligent use of the positive or negative hand is the secret of a good balance. There is, however, one major exception to this rule and we would do well to remember it: in case of a bacterial or viral infection, which is in fact a life itself, never use the right hand first on such areas as this could exacerbate the problem. In such cases always use the left hand.

To stimulate the energies in the body, the method used can be likened to "charging the human batteries". The positive right hand is always applied to the positive right side, i.e. the right hand on the right side (front of the body), and the right hand on the positive left side (back of the body). Also, the negative left hand is applied to the negative right side (back of the body). Never apply too much pressure or rub or massage too firmly; instead, try to use a very gentle touch.

There is no doubt that the energies described above do exist and can influence the healing process of every organ tissue, through direct or indirect contact with the surface area of the human body. This was found to be so by the ancient Chinese more than 2,000 years ago. If you put it to the test you will realise that by using these vibrating centres on the body's surface you will be capable of producing remarkable results. The secret, then, of maintaining the endocrine balance is the involvement of the qualities of body energy. It has been found to be true that conscientious application of these simple techniques can bring rapid relief from harmful tensions. In a similar way reflexology and aromatherapy, especially when using the thumbs, have a far-reaching and penetrating effect on the endocrine balance.

8

Exercises

"YOU CAN'T BE SERIOUS!" is typical of the reaction I have come to expect from patients when I explain that exercise is beneficial during times of stress. Exercise helps to take one's mind off a particular problem, and it also helps to relieve stress. Exercise can also be seen as a means of preventing more widespread damage during possible future attacks. Having acknowledged the importance of physical exercise, we may wish to regard the body as a piece of delicately balanced equipment which has been designed with great technological and scientific knowledge, and consisting of three parts:

an interesting and effective skeletal system, where the bones are held together by ligaments in such a manner as to provide joints. Muscles have been included to introduce motion into these joints and nerves to control their action;

then there is the mind — a gift that makes us different from all other creatures;

the third part can be likened to several extremely delicate processing and manufacturing plants which are contained within the body and designated as the viscera. These processing plants are designed to take in a variety of raw materials and convert them into products to be used by the various components of the manufacturing division.

These three parts, although often separated into areas for the osteopaths, psychiatrists and internists respectively, are actually welded into one total functional unit by the autonomic nervous system. I have already referred several times to the endocrine system, but I have made little mention as yet of its counterpart — the autonomic nervous system. This combination constitutes the great two-way-street by which the three major components of the body are tied into fundamental and functional units. Anything, large or small, which happens in one part, will be reflected in one or both of the other parts. The general attitude among practitioners has been a tendency to limit themselves to two parts of this human machine — the mind or the viscera — while ignoring the mechanical and electrical phase. Yet this tripolarity of existence is very important. Life means movement, which requires as rhythmic a balance as possible.

The human body is made up of atoms and the life force within the body maintains its normal rhythm. The nervous system instigates all the functions of the body, unless the motor system is disturbed, when excessive or deficient action results. If the sensory system is disturbed, pain may result. The sympathetic nervous system, as the superintendent of all bodily functions, establishes the circulation of the blood and other fluids. Man is fundamentally made perfect, but certain influences will lead to deviations in terms of health. By all means separate the disease from the person, but be specific in the treatment of definite and indefinite deviations.

Our mental power enables us to deal intelligently with health factors and anyone who is determined to do so can improve their health, if the time is allowed to put that belief in motion through the laws of nature. Every thought is like sending signals to a reception area of a malleable substance, which receives the signal and creates an impression of that thought. If we realise how unconscious and negative thoughts are able to enter this reception area and leave their impression on this malleable substance, we will recognise that such thoughts simply perpetuate our condition. This is why people slide from bad to worse or, conversely, from success to greater success.

So, within every man and every woman there is a force which directs and controls the entire course of life. It can heal every affliction and ailment to which mankind is exposed. Energy must be allowed to flow. Any energy blockage, including the menstrual problems which constitute our current subject, will trigger further responses. It is important that the right techniques are applied in order to overcome the condition and to this end exercising is a powerful weapon.

Relaxation is also important and no pain relief can be obtained unless relaxation is used as a keynote. Exercise has the effect of stimulating the metabolism and therefore it benefits the entire digestive system, which is often in turmoil before, during or after the menstrual period. Correct exercising is a means of stimulating the flow of oxygen through the whole system into the muscle tissue. Regular, sustained, comfortable exercise will induce a marvellous feeling of well-being.

A long-established Indian principle is that all body fluids correspond to the emotional principle, soft tissue to the mental principle and heart tissue to the spiritual principle. The solar plexus is therefore very important as it is the centre of the hormonal system. It has a highly disturbing effect if it is in a state of tension. Stress always shows from top to toe, but especially in the feet. It is like a telephone switchboard: when the light comes on it shows which line is being called, except it is not actually a line, but a circuit. The pattern must be changed before any response can be felt. Be adventurous and try a different approach. I can assure you that it is not such a silly idea to walk outside barefoot, whether it be in the grass, in the snow or on gravel. Such a simple thing constitutes good exercise, as signals are sent from the feet all through the body and pressure points in the feet will stimulate parts elsewhere in the body.

Another relaxation exercise is a method referred to as "visualisation technique". This must really be considered as one of the easiest forms of exercise and all that is required is for the individual to practise the training of mental discipline and the results will repay you handsomely. The following exercise is quite easy, and very worthwhile as long as the preparatory part is done correctly.

Pre-exercise preparation
Sit down in an easy chair, with your head resting comfortably and your feet placed flat on the floor. Breathe calmly and listen to the sound of your breathing while inhaling and exhaling. Next, take a very deep breath and concentrate on relaxing while breathing out. Do this three times.

Continue by concentrating on the muscles of your body. Begin with the eyes and mouth. Squeeze your facial muscles tightly and then suddenly let go. Feel a wave of relaxation travel down the whole of your body. Consciously relax your neck, then your shoulders, arms, hands, and move further down the body to your stomach, back, upper legs, calves and feet. Having done this, think about being in a place where you would love to be. It could be by a lake, in the mountains, or any holiday spot where you have felt at ease and where you have experienced enjoyment and relaxation. Imagine yourself there and stay with the memory for a couple of minutes.

So much for the preparation; now we come to the actual exercise.

Visualisation exercise
Now we are going to have a look at the illness. With your mind's eye *see* the spinal cord. *See* the blood vessels opening, bringing a flood of healthy blood, rich in vitamins. Consider what these vitamins and minerals mean to the body's defence system, which is largely housed in the spinal cord, and how you are going to benefit from the rich supplies which are constantly replenished.

Now, having completed this mental picture (and you may use your own imagination, as long as you see your illness as *weak* and your bodily defence as *strong*), you are going to see yourself quite strong again. *See* yourself walking along the side of the lake or up the mountain slope, striding out full of vitality. Compliment yourself on doing so well.

Breathe deeply three times and open your eyes.

Do this exercise three times a day: when you wake up in the morning, at lunchtime, and before you go to sleep. Never skip an exercise and make sure you isolate yourself in a quiet and solitary place where you can follow this routine undisturbed. Do not force yourself, it is enough just to *see* it with your mind's eye.

What you are really doing is putting a new (and healthy) programme into your computer. Trust that the new programme is going to work, but do not expect miracles. Prepare yourself to be patient, but rest assured that eventually the effects of the new programme will infiltrate all the body.

Always remember the importance of daily physical exercise, not only because most of us can do with losing a bit of weight, but also because a brisk walk, a bicycle ride, a few lengths in the swimming pool or a game of tennis or badminton are excellent ways of releasing tension. Try not to allow yourself to feel uptight over things which are not under your control to change. When you know your period is due, consider that the body has its own way of dealing with this phenomenon and accept this. If need be, take some extra exercise at this time of the month. But remember, nature will have its way. All you can do is try to understand what is happening in the body and by doing so you may come to accept the body's functions and counteract the symptoms by sensible and positive measures.

Regular exercise not only increases the ability to cope with stress, but it also reduces the risk of developing stress-related diseases. The entire body benefits from exercise largely as the result of improved cardiovascular and respiratory functions.

Some progressive relaxation may be done, which enables you to experience the sensation of relaxation techniques by means of a simple procedure involving the alternation of muscle tension and relaxation.

Concentrate on a specific muscle and contract it forcefully for one or two seconds, before letting go. A feeling of relaxation will then be experienced. Repeat this, progressing to muscles all over the face, neck, shoulders, upper arms, lower arms, stomach, upper and lower legs, ankles and feet — and eventually deep relaxation will creep through the whole of the body. Concentrate on the procedure and reprogramme your body's computer. Tell your innermost self that you feel relaxed and work through the body according to a checklist: forehead, jaws, neck, shoulders, abdomen, etc. Keep telling yourself throughout that you are truly relaxed.

Also remember that it is unwise to cross your legs when sitting in a chair. This can easily block the circulation. If you really feel uncomfortable unless your legs are crossed, which is the case with many ladies, make sure that they are crossed only at the ankles, never at the knees. Elevate your legs as much as possible, day or night, as it is much easier for the heart to pump the blood downwards than it is for the muscles to squeeze the blood up through the veins.

In my book *Water — Healer or Poison?* I pointed out the benefits of hip baths and advised on the correct methods of taking such baths, which can be an important factor when they are used for relaxation purposes. A hip bath should contain sufficient water to cover the buttocks, while the hands and feet should be kept out of the water so that the circulation is stimulated. Remember that it is possible to achieve this effect even in a small tub. Sit in the hot water for a few minutes, switching for a few seconds to cold water, and then return to hot water. The cold water will temporarily cause all the muscles surrounding the bleeding area to contract and cause the veins to function better, while the warm water will provide you with a sensation of comfort. In cases of haemorrhoids or constipation this is also a useful treatment, and one that is cheap and not requiring a great deal of effort, yet providing great relief.

At the end of the day, take some time to do some of the exercises I have mentioned above. You may already know that a good body massage can be most soothing. Failing that, try and spend some time alone and, distancing yourself from what has gone on during the day, work towards obtaining this feeling of relaxation in your own way.

If you feel unusually tense and find it difficult to reach this state of relaxation, you will benefit from breathing exercises. In China I learned about a particular technique for this purpose, known as the "Hara" breathing method. I received countless reactions to this method when my book *Stress and Nervous Disorders* was first published. To this day I remain immensely grateful for having been introduced to this technique and rarely a day goes past that I do not practise it myself in one form or another.

At about four o'clock in the afternoon, the time of day I was born, I sometimes feel a little tired. This, by the way, is an experience which many people feel when the time of their birth approaches. If given half a chance I will excuse myself briefly and lie down on the floor and relax. This becomes easier with practice. My eyes are closed and I relax individual parts of the body until I feel as if my body is sinking deeper and deeper into the floor. Then I place my left hand about half an inch beneath my navel and place the other hand over the top of it. At that point, a magnetic ring on the vital centre of man — "Hara" — has been formed. The Chinese have an old saying that "the navel is the gate to all happiness" and certainly, by creating this circle, one feels very relaxed. Next I breathe in slowly through the nose, filling my stomach with air and keeping the rib cage still. This sounds easier than it is, but you need not worry if this takes a little time to master properly.

Concentrate the mind on the stomach and breathe in slowly. Once the stomach is filled with air, round the lips and slowly breathe out, pulling the stomach flat. This can be done as often as desired. Normally, the sensation after finishing this exercise is either one of complete relaxation and the desire for a nice sleep, or of refreshment and the desire to return to work. I must stress that the breathing should be regular and follow a natural pattern, like a baby's. Sometimes it helps to imagine yourself in pleasant surroundings, for example a colourful garden, admiring the beautiful flowers and inhaling their delicious scent.

Personally, I always find that ten minutes spent therapeutically in this way increases my energy flow dramatically. According to feedback from patients it is also ten or fifteen minutes well spent if one suffers from stress. It helps to restore the life force which then helps the body to respond positively when treated as a whole.

In my capacity as an osteopath I often see patients who suffer from menstrual symptoms. They complain that their neck, shoulders and upper back are the most troublesome areas in the days leading up to or during their actual menstrual period. Very often I advise them to try the following exercise. Stand in front of a full-length mirror, gently rocking back and forth. The knees should be aligned directly over the ankles and the thigh muscles above the knees, gently pulled up. Relax your shoulders in a line extended upwards from the ankles, letting your arms hang loosely by your side. Lift your head upwards from the crown, feeling the back of the neck lengthening. The entire spine is now stretched. Hold the chin at a right angle to the ground. Such a posture will provide relief. The shoulders and neck are usually the keys to all areas of tension. Remember, however, that the neck is delicate and so should always be moved with care.

Our delicate neck has much to endure from the way we tend to treat it. Our shoulders too are always very important and should be held in the correct position. Sit in a basic position, with your arms loosely at your side. Move the shoulders gently forward in a circular movement a few times and then gently backwards. Do this slowly and keep your arms and hands hanging loosely along the sides of the body. This is a marvellous relaxation exercise.

Another shoulder exercise is to interlace your fingers with your hands behind your seat, with your elbows bent and arms relaxed. Exhale and inhale very slowly and gently. Do this several times and if at all possible try and do it rhythmically.

Yet another shoulder exercise is to let your arms hang loosely at your sides. Inhale and slowly raise your shoulders up to your ears. Exhale as you let the shoulders relax, lengthening your neck as much as possible. Squeeze your shoulder blades, and pull them back quite hard as if trying to get them to meet in the middle. Continue to inhale and exhale, and be aware of the space you are creating between your ears and your shoulders, whilst imagining that a heavy suitcase in each of your hands is weighing you down.

For tension in the neck roll your head in a circular movement, five times to one side followed by five times in the opposite direction. Inhale when your head moves upwards from the shoulder and exhale when your chin rolls towards the chest at the opposite side of the circle. Always tip the head gently backwards, but only as far as is comfortable. Exhale as you slowly bring the head down and gently bend it forward.

To relax the upper back straighten your elbows with your hands clasped behind your back stretching towards your buttocks. Gently pull the shoulders back. Inhale as you raise your arms away from the buttocks, keeping them straight. Lift them as high as possible, squeezing the shoulder blades together, which induces a pleasant sensation. Exhale as you lower your arms again, allowing your elbows to bend. Repeat this exercise several times but try to move rhythmically for the best results.

Always remember to let yourself go. The more you relax, the more tension will be released. Tension is extremely tiring and a total waste of energy. If any further breathing exercises are done, take several deep breaths, feel the rib cage moving up and out, and the breathing will gradually become more rhythmical if you learn to let go. Look at yourself as you exercise because the body speaks an important language and tells us quite clearly if we are doing the exercise correctly. When studying yourself in the mirror, you should see a posture with the shoulders held well down from the ears, without stretching the hands too much. Let them hang loosely by the side. Concentrate on your legs, especially the ankles and feet, and try and relax. Tell yourself that you want to relax. Then look at your face and mouth and tell yourself that this gentle activity is a way to help your whole body.

Lately the martial art of shiatsu has become a popular topic of conversation. Shiatsu is not only recognised as a method of relaxation, but is also regarded as being extremely healthy. Many women with menstrual or premenstrual tension have taken courses in this therapy in order to use it as a form of self-help treatment at home. Shiatsu is an old and well-established Japanese relaxation therapy which was introduced into Britain some years ago. It works a little like acupuncture, except that no practitioner is required. The individual can work on the channels of energy that flow through the body by applying pressure on a specific acupuncture point; by doing so it is possible to influence different parts of the body. The benefits of shiatsu are based on medical facts. By pressing a specific point the body can be encouraged to release some of its own natural morphines or painkillers. So, with a relaxed mind and body the restoration of energy will probably make much of the pain and discomfort disappear.

A good practitioner will take sufficient time to go through the entire body to unblock the energy channels, and by doing so, encourage the mind and body to relax. There are many practitioners, self-help groups and professional counsellors that specialise in giving advice specific to the art of relaxation. In the course of my travels in the United States I have met a number of people who are specifically trained to help people to relax and from them I have learned many new exercises. I have been delighted to pass on such newly discovered techniques to many of my patients.

Some of the self-help relaxation techniques I learned about in the United States are especially recommended for women during the menopause. I learned that colour-breathing has traditionally been used for calming the nerves, healing the body and aiding the body's energy field. Thousands of years ago, in oriental spiritual tradition, the body's energy field was accorded great importance. Although these beliefs appear to have been forgotten for some time, it is now once again recognised that the energy field can be related to lights and colours that emanate from the body. This theory has been tested and proved by means of Kirlian photography, which is a method of capturing the light emanations from the body's energy field.

Earlier in this book I outlined a colour code which appears to relate to certain days during the premenstrual period (see page 54). In the colour-breathing technique I learned in the United States it is claimed that different parts of the body appear to emit different colours: red for the legs, orange for the pelvis and intestines, yellow for the solar plexus, green for the heart, blue for the throat, violet for the eyes and the pituitary gland, and white for the top of the head. It is thought that every colour gives energy and strength to that part of the body to which it is thought to correspond.

When a person is calm and relaxed, the human energy field appears radiant, harmonious and colourful. Emotional imbalances such as anxiety, irritability, insomnia and depression (not uncommon during the menopausal period), can easily upset the existing energy field.

This would then create disturbances in its colour and intensity. Therefore colour-breathing, following the steps below, is considered an effective technique to balance the energy field and to calm both mind and body.

Choose a comfortable position, either sitting or lying. Imagine that the earth beneath you is red and that this colour has penetrated deep into the ground. While inhaling slowly, imagine that your body is soaking up this same colour. Visualise the colour creeping up by way of the feet, legs, abdomen, trunk, arms, neck and head. When your entire body has taken on the colour, exhale and slowly expel the red from the lungs.

Slowly repeat this process several times and then proceed to the next step, which involves replacing the red colour with orange. Again, visualise the earth beneath you as strongly coloured, this time orange. Follow the procedure described above, all the time imagining that the body takes on the orange colour. Eventually, having expelled the orange air from the lungs, repeat the exercise with each of the other colours mentioned on page 54.

The next exercise, also specifically recommended for premenstrual tension, requires a little preparation:

Settle in a comfortable position, and for most people this means lying on the back. However, if preferred, the exercise may also be done while sitting up. Comfortable and loose clothes should be worn and make sure that the spine is straight. Your arms and legs should be loosely stretched and never crossed. Concentrate hard while doing the exercise in order to achieve maximum benefit. Close your eyes and concentrate on breathing — in and out, in and out. Concentrating on the breathing pattern makes it easier to shut out the thoughts of tasks that are ahead of you or of nagging problems. Remember that abdominal breathing transports oxygen to all the tissues of the body. It is well known that oxygen is the fuel for metabolic activity, which increases health and vitality. Irregular and rapid breathing depletes our oxygen supply and so devitalises us. Deep breathing helps to relax the whole of the body and simultaneously strengthens the chest and abdominal muscles.

Lying flat on your back, pull your knees up and place your feet flat on the floor, slightly apart. Breathe in and out through the nose.

Inhale deeply, allowing your stomach to relax, letting the air flow into the abdomen. When breathing in deeply, your stomach should rise and your lungs will make your chest swell. Imagine that the air you inhale is filling the body with energy.

Exhale completely, allowing your stomach and chest to collapse. Imagine that the released air disappears, first from the abdomen, and then from the lungs.

A further exercise is specifically designed for those who are aware of tension building up during the day:

Assume a comfortable position with your arms resting loosely palms down on the floor, and practise deep breathing, right into the abdomen.

Tightly clench your fists and hold for approximately fifteen seconds. While doing this, relax the rest of the body, before consciously relaxing the hands. Relax for about thirty seconds before moving on to a different part of the body: the face, shoulders, back, abdomen, legs, feet and toes. Each separate part of the body should be tensed for approximately fifteen seconds and then relaxed. Allow yourself about thirty seconds in between.

During this exercise, concentrate on the actual contraction of the part of the body you are tensing, and maintain that concentration while relaxing. This must also be done with awareness of what is happening. It may require some practice initially, but try to imagine the energy flowing through the whole of the body, leaving the muscles soft and pliable.

When all parts of the body have been tensed and relaxed as described, gently shake your hands, visualising the remaining tension disappearing, seeping out from the extremities, the fingertips and the tips of the toes.

The above are just a few examples of relaxation exercises I was taught in the United States which I have not come across in Europe. It always excites me when I learn about new or unfamiliar methods on my travels, especially when they are recommended, not by practitioners, but by patients.

I will now return to the start of this chapter, where I mentioned the nervous system. The autonomic nervous system will gratefully respond to the relaxation techniques I have described and it is a constant source of amazement how the mind and the body can benefit from such simple and pleasurable methods.

Sometimes it may be helpful to play some soothing, possibly classical, music in the background while performing the above exercises. It is claimed, rightly so, that music softens the heart, and it also has a gentle influence on our moods and our state of mind.

With the knowledge that seven glands make up the endocrine system, which is the most important factor in menstrual problems, we ought to remember that a musical octave has seven basic steps. There should be harmony in colour, harmony in light, and harmony in the body. Music will relax and it can be considered as one of the most powerful healers for women who have a tendency to depression, irritability or aggression at certain times of the month. There can be a terrific change in one's attitude when singing or humming a tune; it will often help to lift the spirit. The wonderful colours that are seen in the rainbow contain the promise that everything will turn out better than we could hope for and our mental attitude is a major factor in the state of our health. This understanding is further confirmation that we must accept responsibility for our health and such acceptance indicates the individual's capability to influence his or her health one way or the other.

9

Reflexology and Aromatherapy

REFLEXOLOGY IS A FORM of treatment which involves massaging all areas of the feet. The feet contain certain reflex areas which relate to every part of the body and these reflex areas are to be found on the soles, the top and the sides of the feet. In fact, the feet as a whole correspond to the whole of the body. By massaging the various areas, a diagnosis can be made of those organs and parts of the body that are out of balance. Areas and organs that are not functioning correctly can be treated by massaging certain areas on the feet, and in this way the body can be returned to good working order.

Similar reflex areas exist in the hands and again these correspond to the whole of the body. The hands can also be used for treatment, although practitioners generally prefer to use the feet for treatment as they are considered more responsive. The feet not only offer a larger area to be treated, but as they are usually protected by footwear, they present a more sensitive area for treatment than the hands. The hands are used when it is difficult or impossible to work on the feet. In general, however, the hands are considered a better area to work on for the purpose of self-treatment.

Thousands of years ago the ancient Chinese practised various forms of medicine that were quite different to those used in the West. The best known of the Eastern treatment methods must be acupuncture, which involves the insertion of needles into certain areas of the body referred to as acupuncture points. These points are situated on lines known as meridians, which are "energy" lines distributed throughout the body. By inserting a needle at a certain point, energy within a meridian can be redistributed, resulting in the correction of the ailment associated with this meridian. Usually the needle is inserted in an area quite distant from the part of the body for which the treatment is required. Yet the treatment will still be effective because the treated area is linked by the meridian line to the problem area.

Reflexology is based on similar theories to acupuncture. Here also it is believed that energy lines link the extremities to various parts of the body and that the whole body can be treated by working on the reflex areas or pressure areas in the feet and hands. I must stress, however, that the energy lines in reflexology are not the same as the acupuncture meridians, but undoubtedly the system is based on the same origins as the ancient Chinese therapies.

In an Egyptian tomb a drawing was discovered, dating back to 2330 BC, in which a person is shown massaging the sole of the foot of another person. We now know that the principles of reflexology were also known to the North American Indians and certain African tribes.

Only a few days before writing this chapter I referred a very depressed patient to one of the reflexologists in our clinic. I tried to explain to her how reflexology works and that this treatment could help to relieve her condition. I may not have made too good a job of explaining the principles to her, because she still appeared sceptical. She asked how administration to the feet would be able to relieve her of some of the severe menstrual symptoms she experienced. I suggested that she should give it a try and then come back afterwards to let me know how she felt. One and a half hours later she returned to my consulting rooms to tell me that she felt renewed. She felt invigorated and wanted to know how long the effects were expected to last and, please, could she book another appointment.

Reflexology and aromatherapy are enjoying an upsurge in popularity, which to me is not surprising. We know that these methods were used diagnostically and therapeutically by ancient civilisations. In the context of menstrual and related problems the beneficial influence of aromatherapy and reflexology are invaluable to the endocrine system.

When thinking about our health in general, we tend to overlook our feet. For the purpose of balancing secretions of hormones from the glands, relaxation, exercise, palpation, massage or manipulation can be applied. The secret of hormonal balance is to balance body energy, and the best method is to use the thumbs of both hands for contact. The thumb is the most important part of the hand for polar energy. It is possible for individuals to administer to themselves, but it is far easier to have these techniques applied by others.

"Zone therapy" is closely related to reflexology. It is believed that this treatment method enables the practitioner to reach the very important centres of energy, called the "chakras". This allows an experienced and well-trained practitioner to improve the body energy balance. Foot exercises and proper care of the feet are always important because the feet are excellent indicators of how the body feels as a whole. It is significant that when people complain of tired feet, it often means that somewhere in the body something is out of balance. The sooner such signals are correctly interpreted and the appropriate treatment applied, the better. It is amazing that certain reflexes in the feet can alert us to the fact that specific organs in the body are under threat or in need of attention. Once the reflexes in the feet have been studied and identified, it is relatively easy to deduce whether the cause of the problem lies in the thyroid, the ovaries, the adrenals or in any of the other organs.

When taking a footbath, use salvia oil or some St John's wort oil. Other excellent oils to use are the lemon and orange oils from the Bioforce range. As is so often the case, we do not appreciate our feet until we become aware that the balance of the body is totally reliant on them and their reflexes, as people who have been unfortunate enough as to lose a foot will be able to tell us.

The feet also have many acupuncture points which are important for the endocrine system. Through these points we are able to influence the energy throughout the entire body, carrying it to the various glands and organs. I have several good friends who are active in the field of reflexology and aromatherapy, and who have conducted thorough investigations as a result of which they are making more and more progress in this science and constantly discovering new aspects. Shirley Price, for example, has written some excellent books on the subject, as has Nicola Hall, and both have spent much time and effort on investigation into the potential benefits that can be obtained using these methods.

All natural therapies have the same aim: to balance the body. Please note that only pure oils should be used for either inhaling or as an addition to the bathwater, and they must *always* be diluted. Generally, these oils have a relaxing effect and sometimes several oils are mixed together or combined with herbs. Indeed, there is an enormous range of different combinations of oils and they can be mixed to suit widely varying purposes. These high quality oils are an essential requirement for achieving the marvellous results possible from aromatherapy and reflexology.

Pure oils, which are extremely potent, prepared for the specific purpose of aromatherapy are recognised as possessing properties which can alleviate stress and depression. To me it is an added bonus when the whole of the plant is used and as such the holistic principle is adhered to. Sometimes specific parts of the herb or plant are isolated and extracted, but I believe it is important that we look at the strength of the complete plant and use this for our oils and remedies.

These pure essential oils used for reflexology work in magical ways. Among my patients I can list quite a number of women with menstrual complaints who are enthusiastic about this treatment and the list of oils or combinations they have used appears endless: basil, bergamot, clary-sage, thyme, chamomile, camphor, geranium, lavender, neroli, frankincense, jasmine, rose, sandalwood, ylang ylang, lemon and pine.

Especially recommended for the purpose of relaxation and for the treatment of depression and painful periods are the following: cajuput, sage, aniseed, chamomile, citrus, juniper, marjoram, melissa, peppermint, rosemary, jasmine and tarragon.

For severe menstrual problems the following oils are suggested: lavender, melissa, neroli, rose, geranium, chamomile and clary-sage.

It is also possible to use all the above herbal oils for gargling or compresses.

A considerable number of publications have appeared on the reflexes of the feet by authors such as Fitzgerald, Bressler, Reilly, Daglish and Lust, to name but a few. Yet my favourite book on this subject must be Eunice Ingham's *Stories the Feet can Tell*. Dr William Fitzgerald, an American ear, nose and throat specialist, noticed that when operating on different patients for the same disorder, some would feel considerable pain, while others would feel very little. His subsequent investigations revealed that those who felt little pain were actually producing an anaesthetic effect on themselves by unwittingly applying pressure to certain areas of the body. Although they may be unaware of the principles of reflexology, people apply this theory in everyday life by such actions as gritting their teeth when in pain, or grasping the sides of the dentist's chair, respectively applying pressure to zones in the jaws or in the hands. By embellishing further on these early theories Dr Fitzgerald was able to identify a system of ten zones in the body; within each zone there is an energy link between certain areas, allowing one area to affect another area in the same zone.

If you imagine a vertical line drawn through the centre of the body, there are five zones on either side of this median line. Each zone relates to one of the digits of the body, i.e. the fingers and toes. The importance of the ten vertical zones throughout the body is that those parts of the body that are found within a certain zone are related to one another by the energy flow within that particular zone. Thus they can affect one another. A striking example of this theory is the fact that kidney trouble may result in eye problems, and this can be explained by the fact that both organs are situated in the same zone.

For some time now I have used these feet reflex areas for diagnostic purposes and for researching into body zones and the occiput. I have had a great degree of success with this method, with the result that patients find greater relief after treatment. In some of my earlier books I have already explained that the head is the positive pole, the feet comprise the negative pole and the hands comprise the neutral area. Only when the whole body is balanced will we have succeeded in the treatment. It may help to compare the body to the battery of a car, which also has a positive and a negative pole, and in the middle of the battery we find the neutral area, where nothing happens. The best part is that we know that positive always looks for negative; negative never seeks positive. So with positive action and positive thought, we can be relieved of menstrual problems.

For centuries now the Chinese and the Indians have used this diagnostic material. It is worth knowing that all the hormonal reflexes can be found in the feet; indeed, the science of endocrinology, which embraces the internal secretions of all the ductless glands, is greatly advanced by this knowledge. Unfortunately, too little credence is generally given to this science and I sometimes wonder if this is because of the apparent simplicity of the treatment methods that relate to the endocrine system. Most people are sceptical about the outcome: why should their feet be kneaded and massaged if they feel a little down in the dumps? Eventually, after they have tried reflexology treatment, they tell you in amazement how other problems, such as corns and calluses, have been cleared up at the same time.

The big toe is an important health indicator. It is possible for a displaced joint, or a bunion, ultimately to cause problems in the head. The big toe reflects the head and contains the reflex areas for several of the endocrine or hormonal glands, which are also represented in the thumbs. A well-trained and qualified reflexologist or aromatherapist, by working on the big toe, can re-establish harmony in the entire hormonal system. The "chakras" or glandular areas are all functional and represent the quality of life which flows from the head down. In fact, these glandular areas connect the upper areas with the lower areas, the positive with the negative principle. This is further enhanced with the use of the hands, which comprise the neutral principle.

The right foot corresponds to the right side of the body and the left foot corresponds to the left side of the body. Similarly, the right hand corresponds to the right side of the body and the left hand corresponds to the left side of the body. The reflex areas are arranged in such a way as to form a small picture of the body in the feet and, to a lesser extent, in the hands. Certain types of diseases and complaints can be helped by this technique alone, but the use of the whole sensory motor technique — using the positive, negative and neutral poles — accelerates recovery and the subsequent improvement is permanent.

As we move on to consider the actual technique applied in various ways on the human body, both anteriorly and posteriorly, we will see that it consists of balancing different areas. The curative effect of this kind of massage has gained increasing recognition and in many parts of the world it is now an accepted part of complementary or alternative therapy.

The thyroid gland reflex area is found in the sole of the foot or the palm of the hand, more specifically at the base of the proximal phalanx of the big toe or thumb. This is the area on the top half of the ball of the big toe or thumb, and the reflex area can be found in both the right and left feet or hands. The thyroid gland produces the hormone thyroxine, which is responsible for stimulating the rate of cell metabolism; it also influences the rate of growth and sexual development.

Under-activity of the thyroid gland in adults causes weight gain, puffiness in the face and eyelids and a slowing down of the metabolic processes resulting in weakness, tiredness and lethargy. On the other hand, an over-active thyroid gland serves to speed up all the body processes, resulting in restlessness, nervousness, irritability, increased perspiration and weight loss. In such circumstances the gland itself may swell and the eyes will protrude. These are all obvious signs of an over-active thyroid gland.

The reflex area for the thymus gland is also found in both feet and hands, again in the big toe or the thumb. The thymus gland plays an important role before the age of puberty in the development of the body's immune system. After puberty the size of the gland decreases and little is known about the exact function of the thymus gland in adulthood, although it is thought that it may still have some influence on the immune system.

The soles of the feet and the palms of the hands also contain reflex areas for the pancreas. This gland is best known for its production of insulin, which controls the blood sugar level. The pancreas is also involved in the digestive processes and it produces substances called pancreatic enzymes which break down food into smaller-sized particles which can be more readily absorbed by the digestive tract. This reflex area is therefore of specific importance in the treatment of patients with diabetes or hyper- and hypo-glycaemia, as well as certain other digestive problems.

Pressure points relating to the kidneys are also found in the soles of the feet or in the palms of the hands. The kidneys lie to the back of the abdomen, with the right kidney being positioned slightly lower than the left kidney. These bean-shaped organs are about 10 cm in size and their function is to separate certain waste products from the blood. After a process of filtration and concentration in the kidneys, urine is formed, which then collects in the bladder. The kidneys form part of the waste-disposal system of the body and the term urinary system includes the kidneys, ureter, bladder and urethra. The right kidney is represented in the right foot or hand, and the left kidney in the left foot or hand.

The reflex areas for the adrenal glands are situated very close to those of the kidneys, slightly above the kidneys' reflexes to the medial side. In the body, too, the adrenal glands are positioned close to the kidneys; in fact, they are placed like small caps on the upper and medial part of each kidney. The adrenal glands produce several hormones, the best known of which is adrenaline. This hormone influences the sympathetic nervous system by preparing the systems of the body to react quickly and efficiently in times of stress.

In view of the subject of this book we should also have a closer look at the ovaries. The reflex areas for these glands are found on the outer side of the foot near the ankle. The right ovary is represented on the right foot or hand, while the left ovary is represented on the left foot or hand. Women possess two ovaries, one on each side of the pelvis, each one being about the same size and shape as a shelled almond. The ovaries constitute part of the female reproductive system and they produce the female germ cells — or ova — from the time of puberty until the menopause. The ovaries also produce the hormones oestrogen and progesterone, which influence the cyclical changes that take place during the production of the ova, unless fertilisation has taken place and the woman has become pregnant.

Well, I have tried in this chapter to give you a brief insight into the art of reflexology and you will now have read enough to realise that this is a topic that deserves much more space than I can afford here. The point I constantly try to make is that many of the old treatments deserve to be resurrected and investigated much more deeply. People have become used to the sophistication of modern orthodox medicine and are usually determined to write off the older treatment therapies with an attitude of "we now know better!" Much of my time is taken up with having to produce contradictory arguments and I am constantly urged to produce evidence in black and white as to how and why these therapies work. Yet the principles underlying these therapies were established centuries ago. I ask you, is it possible to state categorically how energy works? I most definitely believe that we have an awful lot more to learn about the vast area of knowledge that can be captured under the umbrella term "energy". Will it ever be possible to really explain the concept of "energy"? It is time that the medical profession shed their conceit and delved deeper into the knowledge accumulated by our predecessors, and their beliefs, which were developed centuries ago, became the subject of more in-depth studies.

Finally, as an aid to self-help treatment, I would suggest that we always remember that the palm of the right hand contains positive energy, while the palm of the left hand contains negative energy. For now it will have to suffice that we bear in mind the saying: "To know is common, but to know what one should know is very uncommon".

10

Conclusion

ENDLESS ARTICLES have appeared in newspapers and magazines about menstrual and premenstrual tension, sometimes referred to as PMS or PMT, but basically they all deal with the same subject. PMS stands for premenstrual syndrome, while PMT refers to premenstrual tension. The latter is the expression most often used by doctors and medical specialists as it covers a multitude of symptoms.

I am often asked if every woman suffers from menstrual symptoms. Indeed, most women do experience some of the symptoms to a greater or lesser extent. It may only be apparent or recognised in temporary constipation, or it may be more substantial such as swelling of the breasts, bloatedness, irritability, etc. It is my sincere belief that an increasing number of women are experiencing more severe symptoms and the reason for that must be the stress of modern life. It may be the start of a new job, unwise eating habits, spending too much time at the word processor, personal relationships, a bereavement, or moving house. You will understand from the variety listed here that menstrual symptoms can be aggravated by many apparently unrelated influences. We tend to overlook the fact that many aspects which appear unconnected to one's health still affect us in that they are stress-inducing.

Always remember my advice in the section on dietary management, because low blood sugar can have a further adverse effect. Eat regular and wholesome meals. Irritability or aggression may occur as a result of overeating, or because of poor nourishment, i.e. food containing colourings or chemical additives.

Women are often apologetic for the seemingly trivial symptoms that may occur because of menstrual conditions. Please understand that there is no reason to be ashamed, because millions of women are in the same situation. It is part of nature. Yet, having said that, I must stress that there is no need to suffer unnecessarily, because this book contains ample advice on how to relieve these problems. I must point out that nothing is to be gained by being envious of a sister or a girlfriend who does not experience similar symptoms, because that is nature's way. Understand and believe that you can help yourself. Perfect harmony in the hormonal system is most uncommon. Those women who are unaffected by menstrual symptoms ought to consider themselves lucky, because they form a small minority.

In summing up, I must emphasise that copious amounts of coffee or fizzy drinks only give you a very short-term lift. The same goes for alcohol. Do not be satisfied with a quick pick-me-up, because the symptoms will only be exacerbated and return with increased ferocity. It is true that prior to menstruation women often feel more thirsty than usual. If this is the case seek the advice of a doctor or practitioner, because there is no easy cure for it. It is best to drink mineral water, but be careful not to induce a bloated feeling by over-indulging.

By now you will understand what I have been trying to say. There is no simple cure for menstrual symptoms, because it is part of a natural process. By keeping stress to a minimum and by being sensible about food intake and exerc'se, one does what one can, realising that there is no universal cure. It is a condition that should be accepted and by taking positive action in your own way, it can be overcome.

However, one thing is certain and that is that medical research increasingly shows that the health and well-being of menstruating women depends greatly upon their diet and lifestyle. Research has also shown that the diet of many women during their monthly cycle is inadequate. Sometimes it is best to make a new start and to this end I recommend the Rasayana course. This is also known as a "spring-cleansing" programme and it does exactly that. It cleanses the organs in the body thoroughly, paving the way to start a new regime. The Rasayana course will cleanse the liver, the kidneys and the bowels, and this can then be followed by a diet such as the one described on pages 64–5. You will also find it beneficial to use the vitamins, minerals, trace elements, and essential fatty acids as advised earlier. Finally, you may decide to try some of the herbal remedies which have also been mentioned.

It is in fact in our own hands to provide relief. Diet, vitamin supplements, herbal remedies, stress reduction and exercising — that's it in a nutshell. After all, we are only on this earth for a very brief spell, and we have the means at hand to make the best of it and to enjoy life to the full. Just remember how wonderfully we have been put together by our Creator and consider the tremendous activity which takes place at certain times of the month in the female body, and you must agree that this is the most tremendous gift of nature: the ability to reproduce. Tremendous activity takes place in the female reproductive organs every four weeks or so. Just imagine that there are 400,000 egg cells in the ovaries, waiting to be released into the Fallopian tubes. Only one ovum is released per cycle. The unused remainder of these egg cells transfers itself to redundant tissue which will have to be disposed of during the menstrual cycle. After the oestrogen-producing period, i.e. the first half of the cycle, the second phase is reached. What happens during that second period is the reason I chose to write this book. The disturbance that then takes place in the hormonal balance is the cause of the symptoms described collectively under the label of menstrual problems. Having read this book, I hope that you now have the confidence to go and do something about your specific problems.

Do not wish this period of your life to be over, because you have been entrusted with the greatest gift of nature: reproductive capability. This must be treasured and the price women are called upon to pay for that wonderful ability can never be too high. The side-effects attached to this priceless gift can be overcome!

Some degree of emotional stress will often be a problem during the latter part of the menstrual cycle. These emotions are often difficult to identify and they may vary in intensity and timing. Yet, you will agree that some of these natural emotions can be positive and can often give us an extra lift. Try to recognise and understand these emotions and come to terms with them, because they can give you a measure of tranquillity. These emotions are stored in the brain for the next experience and through learning to appreciate and recognise them, you will gratefully accept them in admiration of nature's gift of reproduction.

Each emotion influences the glands of the endocrine system in some way or another, and this is true for the male and female species. Maintaining harmony among these glands requires a delicate balance. From my own immediate family, i.e. my wife and four daughters, I have gained an insight into what happens to a woman during her monthly cycle. This understanding has been added to by findings from discussions with patients. I have met with emotions such as anger, resentment, aggression and sheer and utter frustration.

In this book we have dealt with some of the factors that need to be considered. Did you know that a minor increase in the body temperature may release a substantial amount of adrenaline into the blood? We then must react in some way or another to use this release of hormones. So, to alleviate the initial aggravation and increase stimulation, take your time. There is nothing wrong in what we tell our chldren if they tend to fly off the handle: "Count to ten before reacting!" Learn to differentiate between your emotional limitations and avoid situations that may cause them to arise. Remember that most worries exist only in your own mind, because they will cause a state of anxiety which will use up much of your energy. Try to reason through your emotions and do not bottle them up. When emotional stress becomes too much, do not be afraid to confide in someone. The obvious person in most cases must be your immediate partner, and you may be pleasantly surprised by the reaction and understanding you will find in your husband. Otherwise speak to your mother, your sister, or a good friend and you will realise that she too may experience similar emotions.

Use some of the advice provided in this book to learn to relax. Some women will try to put pen to paper and write a letter to a dear friend, which they will find therapeutic. Do not sit and suffer in silence and work yourself deeper into a tunnel of darkness where it becomes increasingly difficult to see the light. Seek out certain activities which have a soothing or relaxing effect on you: swimming, walking, cycling, playing tennis, gardening, playing or listening to music, sketching or painting. Do something! If persistent worry is allowed to take hold, negative emotions will gain the upper hand. If this tendency is recognised, it can be forestalled.

If you find that there are too many demands on your time, whether it be from the family, your friends or your work, feel justified in being a little selfish. Everyone needs some time to themselves. Times have changed and unless we set aside some time for ourselves, we will not be able to give the family or our work the devotion which is expected from us. The structure of our present society is a lesson to love others, but not to the exclusion of loving ourselves.

It may be difficult to train ourselves in the self-control of our emotions, but as I have explained in relation to the endocrine system, it is a matter of the old homoeopathic principle as stated by Hahnemann: mind, body and soul. The hormones produced and secreted by the endocrine glands to regulate the body processes will also influence our mental stability, our soul, and furthermore these hormones are the factors responsible for irrational changes of mood. During periods of menstrual tension, in particular if some extra sugar is taken to satisfy a sudden craving, the pancreas reacts very quickly and the extra sugar intake will rapidly have an effect on the central nervous system. During such times many women either become hyperactive or lethargic. If this is frequently the case, you may like to consult your doctor to check for underlying diabetic or hypoglycaemic conditions.

Preventive care is the best course to take. The old adage is still as relevant as ever: prevention is better than cure. Why fear the unknown? Before the monthly period appears, women often anticipate it with dread. Worry will not make it disappear, but will only result in increased toxicity. Fear will lower one's vitality. Why not try to accept it as a natural phenomenon, take it in your stride with the help of some of the advice contained in this book, and conclude that the menstrual cycle is but a small price to pay for nature's most valuable gift.

Bibliography

Greet Buchner, *Thee uit eigen Tuin*, De Driehoek, Amsterdam, the Netherlands.

Katharine Dalton, *Once a Month*, Fontana Collins, Glasgow, Scotland.

Dorothy Hall, *What's Wrong With You*.

Nicola M. Hall, *Reflexology — A Way to Better Health*, Gateway Books, Bath, UK.

Eunice Ingham, *Stories the Feet Can Tell*.

Arabella Melville, *Natural Hormone Health*, Thorsons, Wellingborough, UK.

Leonard Mervyn, *Vitamins and Minerals*, Thorsons, Wellingborough, UK.

Michael Murray, *Stress Management*, Vital Communications, Bellevue WA, USA.

Sonia Newhouse, *Complete and Natural Food Facts*, Fontana Collins, Glasgow, Scotland.

Carolyn Reuben and Dr Joan Priestley, *Essential Supplements*, Thorsons, Wellingborough, UK.

Maryon Stewart, *Beat PMT Through Diet*, Ebury Press, London.

Dr Alfred Vogel, *The Nature Doctor: A Manual of Traditional and Complementary Medicine*, Mainstream Publishing, Edinburgh, Scotland.

Index

INDEX